COMPLETE HOME HEALTH GUIDE

BOOK ONE

TREATING YOUR BACK PROBLEMS

By Mary T. Fortney

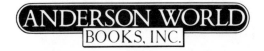

ANDERSON WORLD
BOOKS, INC.

Library of Congress Cataloging in Publication Data

Fortney, Mary T.
  "Treating your back problems."
  (The Complete home health guide; bk. 1)
  1. Backache. I. Title. II. Series.
RD768.F67 1984   617'.56   83-22474
                          ISBN O-89O37-294-2

Each book in the *Complete Home Health Guide* Series is intended for the general health education of the reader. Under no circumstances should any *Complete Home Health Guide* book's information be substituted for the advice and care of a physician when the symptoms of any ailment signal the possibility of a serious condition.

The Editor
Complete Home Health Guides

Book Series design by Kevin J. Moran

Illustrations by Faye Castelli and Kevin J. Moran

Cover art: Michaelangelo's Drawing: For Libyca

Photography by David Keith and Rebecca Colligan.

Models appearing in photos throughout the book are, in alphabetical order:
Theresa Alleaume, Mary M. Cowan, Laura L. Ricco and Robyn Rollins.

Anderson World Books, Inc.
1400 Stierlin Road, Mountain View, CA 94043

CONTENTS

Many thanks to the following who were so helpful in contributing to this book:

From the Palo Alto Medical Foundation:
    Frederick L. Behling M.D.
    Dave Blanchard
    Walter M. Bortz M.D.
    Melvin C. Britton M.D.
    Myron Gananian M.D.
    Rosalind Hawley
    Oakley Hewitt M.D.
    Joan Jack
    John Johnson
    Tami King
    Elston Rothermel D.P.M.
    Robert B. Shelby M.D.
    Jay Thorwaldson

From the Palo Alto YMCA:
    Stephanie Weidert

From the Alexander Technique school:
    Edward Avak, Menlo Park

INTRODUCTION

Mention back problems at a social gathering and the floodgates open.

Everyone immediately has stories to tell. The man recently returned from Europe is still bitterly complaining about missing Munich completely. His back acted up and he had to stay in bed. All he saw of that fascinating city was his hotel room.

A housewife says her husband has to do the vacuuming. It absolutely destroys her back to have to push the vacuum cleaner.

A mother tells about her 35-year-old daughter who has had two back operations. Neither was successful and the daughter suffers continual pain.

A runner who overdid on training for a marathon chimes in with his sad story. His back gave out just before the big race so all his training was in vain.

And someone usually mentions a friend who just bent down to pick up a piece of paper and his back froze in that position.

The stories go on and on. It's a fine way to bring a sense of community into a group. There's a feeling of shared suffering and a common bond of back problems.

But it reflects the unhappy statistics that as many as 80 percent of Americans — or eight out of 10 people — suffer back problems sometime or other in their lives.

An estimated 75 million Americans have recurring back problems. Two million aren't able to work and another five million are partially disabled.

Federal statistics indicate the back is the reason for 31 million visits annually to private physicians. There are other economic costs, too, besides medical bills. Back pain causes 93 million days of work to be lost each year, and back problems tied to job injuries account for $10 billion a year in workers' compensation.

Back problems have been around since man began walking upright, and probably before. X-rays of Egyptian mummies reveal the Pharaoh wrapped inside suffered from an aching back.

Hippocrates, the Greek physician often called the father of medicine, lived in the fourth century before the birth of Christ. Yet he already had devised a method to treat back pain with traction. His system involved having the patient lie on a board. Ropes were tied to the upper and lower parts of the body and a winch tightened them, stretching the spine.

Hippocrates' procedure was primitive, but more sophisticated forms of traction, based on the same principle, are still in use.

Shakespeare, too, was well aware of back problems. In listing diseases in "Troilus and Cressida," he names "loads of gravel i' th' back" and "sciaticas."

Throughout history, back problems have cut across all classes of society. They strike everyone — the farm laborer, the city worker, the rich and the poor.

The late President John F. Kennedy popularized rocking chairs, his way of seeking relief from back pain. Author Ernest Hemingway wrote standing up to ease nagging back pain. Even glamorous movie star Elizabeth Taylor has had bad bouts with a back problem.

Why are there so many sufferers?

A main reason is the sedentary life we lead.

7

Stop and think of the two technological advances that have had the greatest impact on our lifestyle. You're correct if you guessed the automobile and the television. And what do people do while driving a car or watching television? Right again. They sit.

Sitting, according to the experts, is about the worst thing you can do for your back.

Never before have so many people sat so much — and their backs are showing the effects.

Among physicians, two categories of specialists have the most back problems — psychiatrists and radiologists. Psychiatrists sit all day as they spend 50-minute hours with their patients. Radiologists have back problems for a different reason. They must wear heavy lead aprons to protect their bodies from radiation. The apron pulls their spine out of position and makes them prone to back problems. Being overweight has the same effect and, of course, obesity is another characteristic of modern society.

While people may be sedentary, they aren't relaxed. There is always something to do, somewhere to go. People are harried and beset with anxieties, worries about their job or concern for the future of civilization in a nuclear age. Stress also is a major factor in back pain.

All this may sound depressing, as if back problems have always plagued mankind and nothing can be done.

That's wrong. Although back problems have baffled the medical profession for centuries, recent advances have contributed new knowledge.

Many of these gains were made possible by the development of the CAT scan, a new X-ray procedure that produces an image of the back showing soft tissues as well as the bony vertebrae. For the first time, doctors finally were able to get a clearer idea of how the disks, the cushiony pads between the vertebrae, function. That's been a major boost to a better understanding of the reasons for back pain.

The philosophy of treating back problems currently is in a state of transition. Before, it was thought perhaps 80 percent of back problems were due to weak muscles. Patients were treated first for acute symptoms, then given exercises to do to strengthen muscles in their backs, abdomens and legs. Everyone was given just about the same exercise routine.

New insights have changed that stereotyped treatment approach. Today, there's more of a realization that back problems are caused more by disks pressing on nerves than by weak muscles.

Exercises are still prescribed, but they are designed to meet individual needs and with a greater appreciation of how the spine functions.

Even more exciting is a trend toward self-help, toward treating your own back. This trend recognizes the fact that the doctor can't cure your back without your help. Your daily life, how you move, sit and stand, how you sleep, all affect how your back functions. Correct posture, proper lifting techniques, attention to the way you sit can mean the difference between an aching back and a comfortable pain-free life. Attention to these details can help prevent back problems.

It may still be true that "once a back patient, always a back patient," but following proper back habits can do much to make you more comfortable. For the person who so far has been free of back pain, following these precepts can help prevent problems.

Today, the prognosis for back problems is better than it's ever been before.

ONE:

A QUICK QUIZ ON BACK HEALTH

Are these statements true or false?

1. The doctor confirms what your aching back told you. You have a severe back problem so of course that means surgery.

2. The doctors say you have a slipped disk. That means the disk has slipped out of place from between the two vertebrae.

3. You have a pain in the side of your back. Obviously, it's caused by a back problem.

4. Your leg aches and sometimes your toes feel numb. There must be something wrong with your leg.

5. X-rays show degenerative changes in your spine. This means you're a prime candidate for back problems.

6. Every morning when you arise, your back is stiff but it gets better after you've been up a while. You're only 25, so it must be nothing important.

7. People say strong abdominal muscles are important in preventing back problems. You probably should start doing sit-ups daily.

8. You have been suffering pain in your neck. It's probably a disk problem.

9. You have flat feet, but of course that has no connection with your back pain.

10. You've had back problems for a long time and are resigned to accepting the fact that nothing can be done to help you.

Here are the answers.

1. False. Although the typical reaction of most patients is to conclude a diagnosis of back problems automatically leads to surgery, actually only a small percentage of patients need an operation.

2. False. The term "slipped disk" is a misnomer. The disk is still in place but what's happened is that a bit of the jelly-like center has protruded. A herniated disk or a ruptured disk means the same thing.

3. Probably false. There are many other problems that show up as back pain. Your pain might be caused by the kidneys.

4. False. Undeniably, you do have leg problems but the ache doesn't start there. It originates in the spine, where pressure on the sciatic nerve causes pain to radiate down the leg.

5. False. Every middle-aged or older person shows changes as the spine wears with age, but there appears to be little correlation between these degenerative changes and back pain.

6. False. It's very possible the morning stiffness is a first sign of ankylosing spondylitis, a form of spinal arthritis that most frequently affects young males.

7. True. Good stomach muscles do help avoid back problems. But unless you do the sit-ups properly, you may be harming yourself more than helping. The old-fashioned sit-up where you touched your toes is out. The preferred way now is to lie on the floor, knees bent, and raise the head and shoulders off the floor.

8. Probably false. More likely it's due to tension. Most of the problems in the neck and upper spine are caused by muscle tension. Disk problems are more often located in the lower back.

9. False. Podiatrists find flat feet are a factor in back problems. Putting an arch in your shoe may very well alleviate the pain.

10. True. Some patients, even ones who have had several back operations, may never escape back pain. But, luckily, you may fall in with the great majority, who with the support of an interested doctor and with the willingness and self-discipline to follow self-help routines can live comfortably, even with a bad back.

10 EASY WAYS TO BACK HEALTH

1. Stand correctly, with head high, shoulders straight, a slight curve in the lower back, knees slightly bent and weight balanced on your feet.
2. Sit correctly, maintaining the natural curve in your lower back with a cushion or rolled-up towel.
3. Take frequent breaks. Every hour, change your activity, especially if you've been sitting. Walk around for a few moments.
4. To realign your spine, especially after sitting or bending forward, place your hands at the small of your back and bend your back backwards, or get on the floor and do a

press-up. (Lie flat on the floor, face down. Place your hands under your shoulders and press the top half of the body up, arching your lower back. Try to fully extend your elbows and let your back sag. Hold for a few moments, then return to starting position.)

5. Lift correctly. Don't tackle a weight that's too heavy, keep the object close to your body and do the lifting with the leg muscles rather than with your back.

6. Women, especially, should be sure to wear the proper shoes. High heels may be sexy but they throw your back out of balance and put an added strain on it.

7. Sleep the right way — on a bed with a firm mattress, preferably lying on your side with the top leg bent and the bottom leg straight.

8. Keep your weight down. Extra pounds put more strain on your back.

9. Keep physically fit. The better muscle tone you have, the less likely you'll suffer from back problems.

10. Relax. Tension and tight muscles aggravate back problems.

Stand correctly

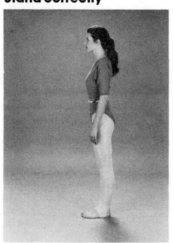

Head high, shoulders straight, slight curve in lower back, knees slightly bent, weight balanced.

Take walking breaks

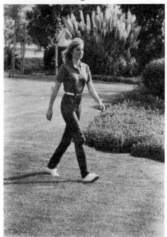

Take frequent breaks, especially if sitting for long periods. Change your activity and walk around.

Bend backwards

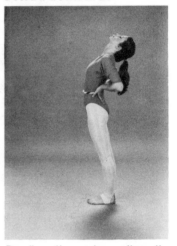

Realign the spine after sitting or bending forward: Place hands at small of back and bend backwards.

Lift correctly

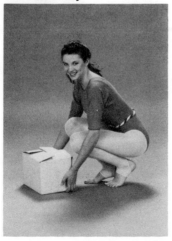

To lift correctly, don't tackle too heavy a weight and keep the object close to your body.

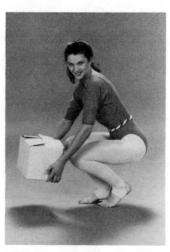

Lifting with leg muscles rather than with your back and keep back straight.

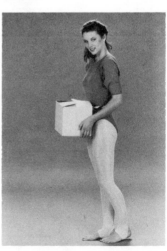

When holding the object in the standing position, keep the back straight.

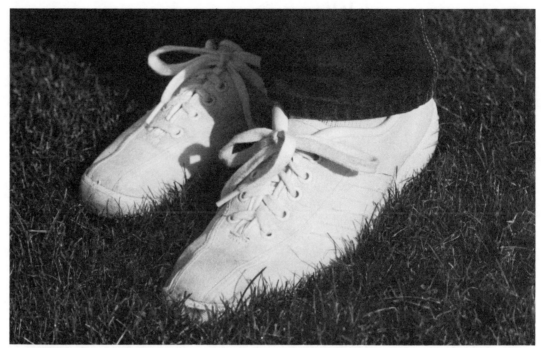

Avoid footwear that throws your back out of balance and puts strain on it. For leisure time, a comfortable pair of sneakers is a good choice.

Stay fit

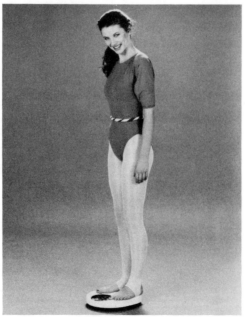

Keep your weight down to avoid adding further stress on the back.

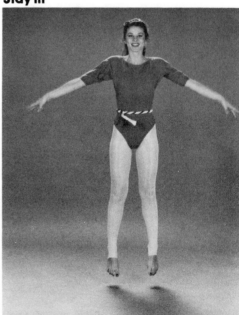

By maintaining good muscle tone through a fitness program, it's less likely you'll suffer from back problems.

TWO:

THE BACK: AN ENGINEERING MARVEL

Have you ever watched a toddler stacking wooden blocks? He's not too adept yet and places the blocks off center. Instead of being a solid stack, the pile curves this way and that.

In a very simplified way, that curve describes the human spine. It is essentially vertebrae — or blocks — stacked one on top of the other, not in a straight line but in an S-shaped curve.

But the spine isn't a simple structure. It's a complicated mechanism that must provide strong support for the body, yet be flexible enough to bend. Not only that, but it serves as a conduit for the spinal cord and as a base for nerve roots that transmit sensations to all parts of the body.

Rather than being surprised at the amount of back problems prevalent in the world, one can only wonder there aren't more. How many man-made machines could function for up to 75 to 80 years or more and have as few breakdowns as the human spine?

BUILDING BLOCKS: THE VERTEBRAE

The spinal column or backbone starts at the base of the skull and ends at the coccyx (the tailbone), actually a vestigial tail. It's the only bone in the body that has no function.

The building blocks are bones called the vertebrae. Usually there are 33, but occasionally the number will vary by one or two.

The vertebrae are named for the regions in which they are located on the spine. Beginning at the top, they are the cervical (through the neck), the thoracic (at the chest level in back), the lumbar (the low back region), the sacral (at the base of the spine) and the coccygeal (in the tailbone).

The five sacral and four coccygeal vertebrae are called false or fixed vertebrae because they are joined together in the adult to form two bones: the sacrum and the coccyx. The sacrum is a roughly triangular-shaped bone connecting the spinal column to the pelvis.

The 12 vertebrae in the thoracic section have limited motion; back problems are rarely located in this region. The seven vertebrae in the cervical region and the five in the lumbar section are notorious trouble spots.

The vertebrae aren't just simple squares of bone, although they do serve as the building blocks of the spine. Instead, they are intricately formed and shaped to fulfill their function in the spinal column.

Each vertebra is composed of two essential parts: the ventral segment (or body) of the vertebra and the vertebral arch (or neural arch). The body, the largest part of the vertebra, is roughly cylindrical in shape. Its surfaces are roughened for the attachment of the intervertebral disk. The vertebra is roughly bean-shaped — convex in front and flattened behind. The flat area forms the front part of the canal through which the spinal

Front view of spine   **Side view of spine**

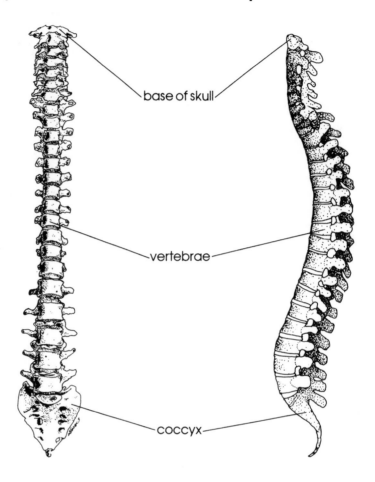

base of skull

vertebrae

coccyx

cord and nerve roots pass. The vertebral arch surrounds the rest of the canal providing a bony protective ring around the spinal cord.

At the back of the spine, the vertebral arches are joined to the arches above and below by small facet joints. One facet joint is located on each side at each level so that each pair of vertebrae are connected by three joints, one between the vertebral bodies and two between the arches.

These are synovial joints, much like the joints in the arms and legs. A lubricant known as synovial fluid allows the joint surfaces to move against one another. Their function is to guide the direction of movement of the spine.

The role of facet joints in back problems is better understood now. They may cause pain by getting out of position or because of arthritic changes.

Each of the vertebrae can move only slightly in relation to its neighbors, but this limited motion still allows enough flexibility for the back to bend. Although all the vertebrae are essentially the same, they vary in size. The cervical vertebrae, bearing only the weight of the skull, are the smallest, shaped so they allow a considerable range of motion. The thoracic vertebrae are middle-sized and provide a transition from the small cervical vertebrae to the large lumbar vertebrae in the lower back.

Vertebral disks. Cushioning the vertebrae are the disks, which physicians at the Palo Alto (Calif.) Medical Foundation describe to their patients as being like jelly doughnuts. The comparison does give a graphic image of what a disk is like. Imagine the vertebrae as building blocks interspersed with jelly doughnuts and the complex structure of the spinal column begins to be understandable.

The disks, although they contain no nerves and can feel no pain, are the cause of much of the agony endured by back sufferers.

Disks are cushions of tissue between the vertebrae, and like vertebrae, are bean-shaped to allow room for the spinal cord to pass through the spine. The disk provides a springy cushion between the vertebrae that can flatten under weight and give with bending and twisting.

It consists of two parts, an outer ring called the annulus fibrosus and a center called the nucleus pulposus.

The nucleus is a jelly-like substance that can be squashed and altered in shape. It is enclosed by the annular ring and by the vertebrae above and below it.

The nucleus of the disk contains large molecules called proteogylcans that are constantly trying to suck in water and swell. The nucleus has a high water content, ranging from as much as 88 percent at birth to 70 percent in old age. The capacity of the nucleus to swell is greater in the lumbar region than in the other parts of the spine.

Normal disk

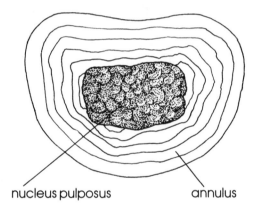

nucleus pulposus   annulus

A normal disk acts as a shock absorber between the bony vertebrae.

Ruptured disk

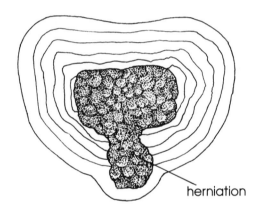

herniation

A disk ruptures when the pulpy body in the center protrudes.

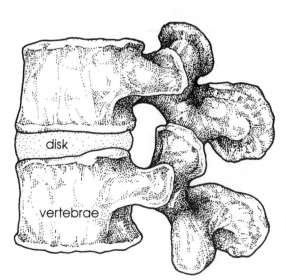

disk

vertebrae

Properly spaced lumbar vertebrae on normal disk.

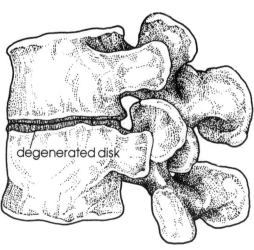

degenerated disk

When disk degenerates, pressure is exerted on nerve roots exiting from spine.

When a person is sitting or standing, compression on the disks may cause fluid loss. At night, when the body lies horizontally in bed, the swelling process is able to take place. That's why people are slightly taller in the morning than they are at night.

The same process caused problems for the early astronauts before the situation was understood. Space suits were individually designed and fitted, but at first the fact that weightlessness would allow the disk nuclei to absorb water and expand was not considered. The astronauts, who may have grown a couple of inches in height after several days of weightlessness, suddenly found their perfectly-fitted suits too short for them.

The annulus fibrosus, the ring surrounding the jelly-like center, is composed of strong strips of collagen fibers arranged like the layers of an onion but crossing at right angles for added strength. The fibers are actually stronger than a steel wire of the same diameter. That strength is essential. The annulus ring may give slightly when pressure put on the spine causes the nucleus to be squashed, but it does not break. When a split or tear occurs, the jelly-like nucleus may leak out. This condition is what's called a slipped, herniated, prolapsed or ruptured disk.

The strength of the annulus fibrosus and the give of the jelly-like center make it possible for the spine to bend forward and backward. Twisting movements are more difficult and put more stress on the disk. For this reason, some back problems will arise after a person twists awkwardly, perhaps to pick up a pencil or climb out of an automobile.

The spinal column is more than an arrangement of bones, vertebrae and disks to support the human body in an upright fashion. It also serves as a conduit for the spinal column and as a base for nerves that lead from the spine to the rest of the body.

The back is closer to our brain and our mind than any other organ of the body. Perhaps for this reason, there is a greater emotional aspect to back problems than with other illnesses.

Bend forward correctly

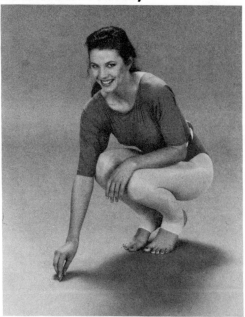

Never twist over awkwardly to pick up something, like a pencil. The correct forward bending motion is to bend the knees and keep the back straight.

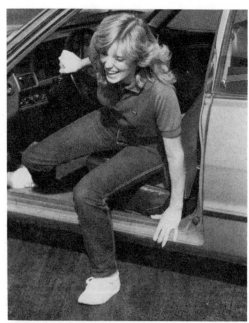

Twisting around and supporting yourself on only one leg to get out of a car increases the chances of a disk problem.

Disk under different pressures

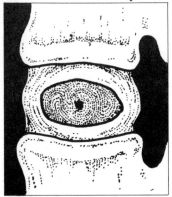

With spine in neutral position.

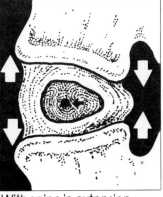

With spine in extension.

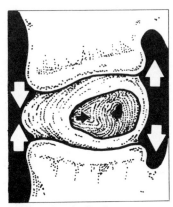

With spine in flexion.

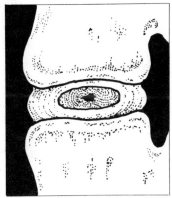

Compression loading.

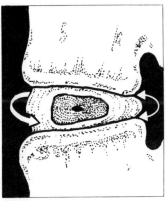

Posterior compression loading.

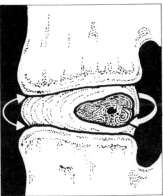

Anterior compression loading.

The spinal cord. The spinal cord begins at the base of the brain and continues down through the neural (or vertebral) arches of the vertebrae. It ends at about the junction of the first and second lumbar vertebrae at the top of the lower back. As it passes down through the vertebrae, nerve roots separate off at every level, emerging through a passageway in the vertebrae called the foramen — the reverse image of thousands of tiny tributaries flowing together to make one giant river. In the back, the tributaries — or nerves — break away from the main river — the spinal cord — to carry nerve impulses to all parts of the body.

Because nerves are so inextricably a part of the back and back problems, often a tingling or numbness of nerves in the feet or hands may signal a problem in the spine.

Sciatica is an example of this kind of nerve pressure — a pain caused by pressure on the sciatic nerve as it leaves the spinal cord. This nerve is the biggest of all nerves, branching throughout the lower body and legs. Pressure on the nerve can be caused by a herniated disk or by osteoarthritis of the spine.

Muscles and ligaments. Helping to hold the spine upright and in place are ligaments and muscles. Bands of strong ligaments encase the vertebral bodies and connect the vertebral arches. The ligaments provide a protective sheath, yet are flexible enough to accommodate the spine's movements.

Further stabilization is provided by powerful muscles attached to the vertebrae, the pelvis and the back of the chest wall. About 140 muscles are attached to the spine to

The nervous system

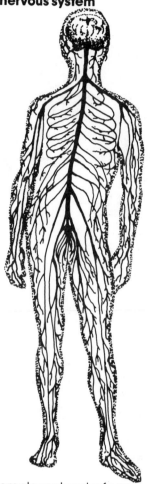

A complex network of nerve cells and fibers travels throughout the body.

The sciatic nerve

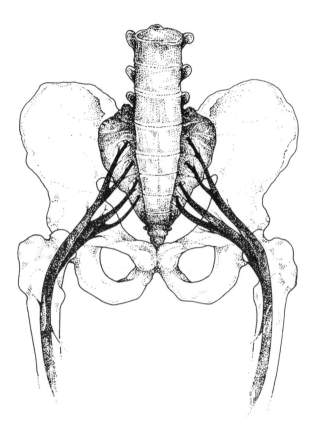

The sciatic nerve is the largest in the human body.

keep it under control. One British writer compared the stabilization of the spine by muscles to the stays on a sailboat which stiffen and stabilize the mast. During any exertion, the muscles contract, stiffening the spine so it can perform its function.

By any reasonable standards, that combination of vertebrae, disks, muscles, nerves and ligaments should be sufficient, and certainly complicated enough to satisfy the most creative designer.

Curves. A straight spine wasn't good enough to meet all the demands put upon the back. Curves had to be added for better shock absorption and flexibility.

The spinal curves have the appearance of a very flattened S-curve. They begin with a slight curve in the cervical or neck region, then curve slightly outward in the thoracic region. Then there's a more defined inward curve in the lumbar or lower-back region, moving out again in a pelvic curve ending at the point of the coccyx.

The thoracic and pelvic curves are called primary curves because they alone are present in the fetus. The other two are secondary curves, developing after birth.

The cervical curve develops when the infant is able to hold up its head and sit upright. The lumbar curve doesn't appear until after the infant begins to walk.

The curves complement each other. The convex thoracic curve is balanced by the concave neck and lower-back curves. They help to give flexibility to the back, yet maintain the center of gravity of the body in a straight line above the ankles.

The concave curves are where most back problems are centered, particularly at the level of the fifth and sixth cervical vertebrae and the fifth and sixth lumbar vertebrae.

Muscles of the back

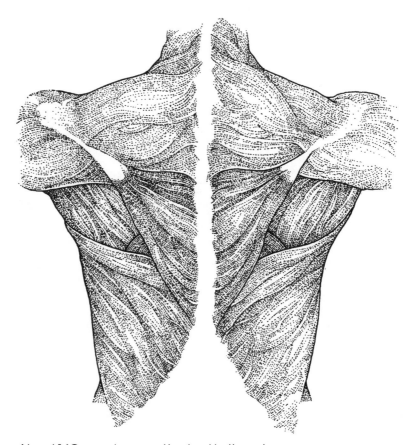

About 140 muscles are attached to the spine.

Because of the curves, the vertebrae aren't stacked straight up on each other. As long as the concave curve is maintained, the pressure of body weight squashes the disk forward away from the nerve canal. Eliminating the concave curve by over-straightening the back or by bending forward creates a greater risk of painful pressure against a nerve, as the nucleus of the disk is pushed backward into the sensitive area. That is the biggest flaw in an otherwise well-designed backbone.

The spinal column works very well in four-legged animals. Although animals do have back problems, particularly the low-slung dachshund, they're minor compared with human back problems.

The spine of a four-footed animal hangs much like a suspension bridge supported by the four legs. The bands of ligaments lie below the spine, helping to support the vertebrae and disks. The spinal cord and nerves lie in a protected canal at the top of the backbone where they are least likely to be exposed to pressure.

Put the same backbone upright and the picture changes.

Upright, the sensitive nerves and spinal cord are at the rear of the spine. Every forward-bending motion is likely to press the cushiony disk against a nerve or nerve root.

Although there is no concrete evidence yet, there is speculation that perhaps genetic influences are a factor in back problems. A person born with a narrow nerve channel or perhaps thinner bony walls in the vertebrae may be just a bit more susceptible to back problems.

That's the picture of your spine. Think a moment about what happens as you sit, the weight of your body pressing down on the disks and vertebrae. Or when you bend, all those vertebrae and disks and nerves acting in unison. The next time you lift a heavy weight, be conscious of the added stress on your spine.

Remember, that spine, with all its parts, must function for your lifetime. It may wear out a little and may cause some pain, but for most of us, it does its job remarkably well.

The spine in four-legged animals

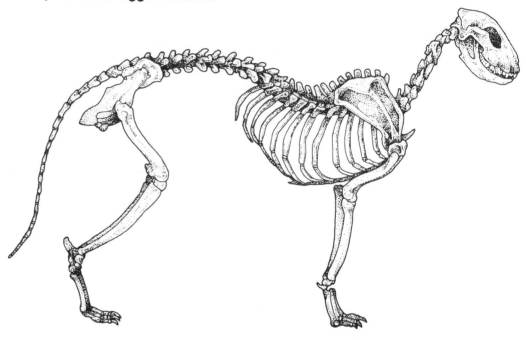

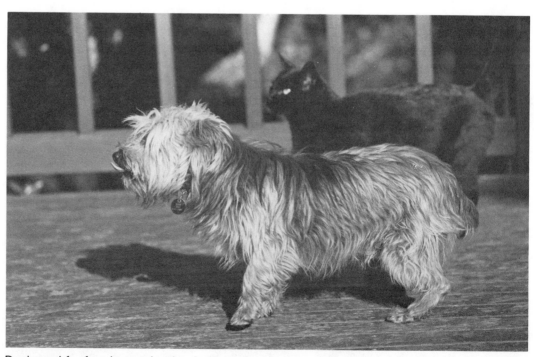

Designed for four-legged animals, the spinal column hangs like a suspension bridge between the legs.

THREE:

BACK PROBLEMS: UNIVERSAL AND UNIQUE

Who gets back problems?

Probably not the Masai warrior in Africa, although no health statistics are available on him. His lifestyle doesn't produce back problems. Most of the time is spent roaming the plains of Kenya, herding cattle. He sits very little and when he does, he squats rather than sinking into an easy chair.

The people who get back problems are the Americans and Europeans who have adopted wholeheartedly the modern lifestyle. Technology is great and has done wonderful things for mankind, but it's done terrible things to man's back.

Henry Ford built the Model-T and cars became an integral part of life. The first Model-T, with its stiff, straight seat, wasn't so bad for the back, but look at the soft, cushioned seats in today's streamlined cars. They're attractive to look at but not the kind of seats that keep a back healthy. Problems are created particularly when people sit for hours, driving their cars or recreational vehicles miles and miles along freeways without stopping.

Sitting is bad for backs because of the pressure it causes on the spine. An experiment conducted in Sweden measured the pressure exerted on disks in the spinal column during different physical activities. The lowest pressure was when the volunteer subject was lying down. Higher pressures developed when the subject was standing or carrying heavy objects. The highest pressures were when sitting, bending forward and carrying a heavy weight. Sometimes the total load on the disk amounted to about a third of a ton.

CURSE OF THE SEDENTARY LIFESTYLE

Think how much of your day is spent sitting. You arise from bed, sit while eating breakfast, then sit while driving to work or on the commute train. Then you sit in your office until lunch, sit while eating lunch, go back to your office for an afternoon of sitting, then it's home to sit during dinner. The day ends with a final sitting session in front of the television set.

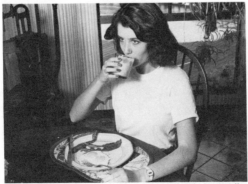

Today's modern sedentary lifestyle calls for a great deal of sitting, starting with a seat at the breakfast table.

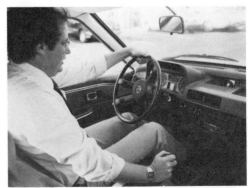

Then, sitting in a car (or train) on the commute to work at the office.

21

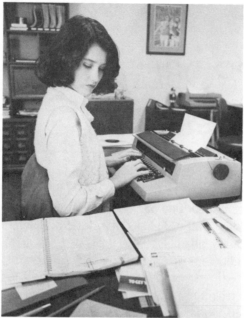

Sitting at your desk in the office, perhaps at a typewriter.

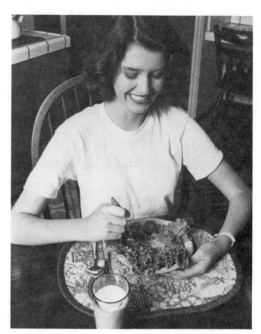

Back to your seat at the lunch table.

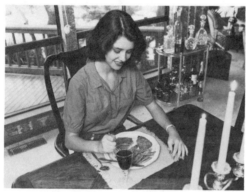

More sitting at the office and on the return commute before you sit to eat dinner.

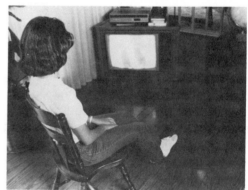

Then, of course, sitting to watch television, or to read before going to bed.

That's what is called a sedentary lifestyle, one that too many Americans practice. It leads to obesity, a further strain on the back.

Then there's the tension of our modern lifestyle. Everyone always seems to feel pressured by time, to be in a constant hurry. We may only sink into a chair to sit for a while after arriving somewhere, but we're still in a hurry to get there.

And there are the anxieties of nuclear weapons, war in the Middle East, disputes in Central America. All contribute to a feeling of stress. When those pressures are combined with a driving sense of ambition, it's even worse for back health.

A prime example is the Hawaiian hotel magnate who returned to a California town for his high school class reunion. He had everything. He was still young and good-looking. His wife was both attractive and loving. But he had something else, too — an agonizing backache that forced him to sit gingerly on the edge of a chair. Instead of being able to enjoy his success and the class reunion, he was in misery.

Back problems are so ubiquitous they can be called a universal affliction, ranking second only to headaches. Back problems can strike at anyone, young and old, poor and rich.

An article in the medical journal, "Spine," reports up to 80 percent of the adult population in Western countries have at some time suffered from lower-back pain. About half that number suffer occasional pain and one quarter of the patients with lower-back pain have consulted a doctor about their problem.

The socioeconomic impact is enormous. It's estimated $14 billion is spent each year treating back problems and paying compensation to workers off the job because of their backs.

Laborers who must lift heavy objects might appear to be the prime candidates for back problems and they do have their share. But back pain hits the housewife and secretary, too, as well as the truck driver and the bank executive.

Men and women are affected about equally. Young people have problems, too, because of congenital abnormalities in their spine. One leg may be shorter than the other or they may have an arthritic-type disease.

The young mother who's hefting a growing infant in and out of his crib also may develop problems.

For most people, back problems begin in their 30s while they are settling down to a sedentary lifestyle. The back begins to age then. Man's original life span was much shorter than it is now; 40 was once considered a good old age. Today, 70 or even 80 years is a reasonable life span. And as people move into their 40s and 50s, more of them are in their doctor's offices, complaining about their backs.

It's often hard to zero in on what back problems cause the complaints. The pain is hard to describe and even harder to diagnose. Some people suffer only slightly, perhaps a stiff back after a Sunday spent gardening. Others undergo several back operations and live in constant torture from the pain.

What is incapacitating for one person may be waved aside by another. Many people are tough enough to live with a recurring back problem. Others rush to the doctor at the first twinge.

EACH CASE IS DIFFERENT

Individuality seems to be the hallmark of back patients. Of course, there is a common complaint — their back hurts. But the causes of the problem and the attitudes of the patients are so different, each person presents his own case.

With other diseases such as cancer, there are support groups. Patients get together to share their problems. With Alzheimer disease or early senility, there are support groups for the families of patients.

The back patient goes it alone, except for informal sharing of complaints with friends over coffee or cocktails. The back patient's family struggles along, too, without outside support.

While back problems are traumatic for the patient, they also can wreak havoc on the rest of the family. A wife may be denied sex because of her husband's bad back. A son may miss the fun of contact sports because his dad is afraid the youngster's back will go out. A man may have to do the housework while his wife lies in bed, having been prescribed bed rest for her bad back.

One of the problems in dealing with back complaints is that it is often hard to determine the exact cause of the problem. Even with the best medical evaluation, it's often difficult to get an accurate diagnosis, particularly of lower-back pain. Estimates indicate from 20 to as much as 85 percent of all lower-back pain cannot be traced to a definite cause.

In ancient times, people thought back pain sufferers were possessed by demons. A witch doctor would be called in to get rid of the demons and the patient would recover. Today, the modern physician must determine which of more than 100 different diagnoses might be causing the problem.

The pain may be caused by a congenital defect in the spine, by a simple muscle strain or by degenerative changes in the intervertebral disks. A facet joint may have been injured and is now inflamed. The problem may not even be in the spinal column. Sometimes a backache is a symptom of cancer or of gynecological problems, such as a tipped uterus. The physician must plow his way through all these possibilities to find the cause, likely a combination of factors.

TESTS AND TREATMENTS

The tools available for diagnosing back problems are still relatively few, even in this technological age. X-rays can be taken of the spine, but they tell nothing about the soft, cushiony disks separating the vertebrae. X-rays, however, can be used to determine if there are changes in the bony parts of the spine. That isn't always a help, because often there is little correlation between the state of the vertebrae and the condition of the patient.

Two major tests, the myelogram and the CAT scan, can be used to diagnose problems in disks.

In a myelogram, a needle is inserted into the spinal column and a fluid that shows up on X-ray is injected directly into the vertebral canal, filling the space immediately behind the vertebral bodies and the intervertebral disks. Any obstruction, such as from a protruded or herniated disk, blocks the flow of the dye, revealing where the disk bulges.

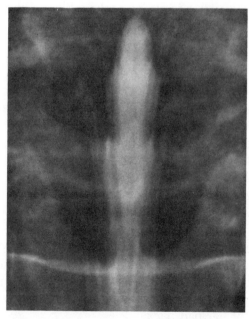

In a normal myelogram, water-soluble fluid fills up space behind vertebral bodies and intervertebral disks. Photo courtesy of Stanford University Medical Center.

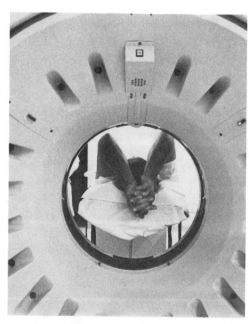

The patient is placed inside the CAT scanner through its "gantry" and holds his arms over his head.

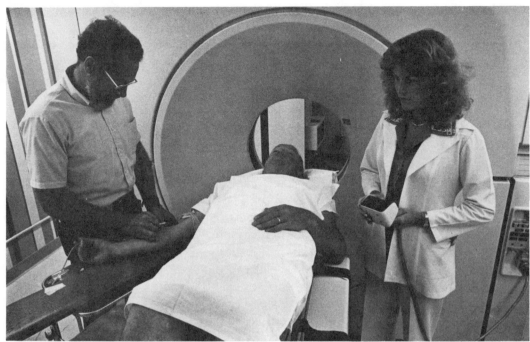

For a Computerized Axial Tomography (CAT) scan, a patient is injected with iodine contrast material. CAT scan photos by Warren Hukill, Palo Alto Medical Foundation.

The myelogram used to be a dreaded, painful procedure. Now a water-soluble fluid is used instead of the former oily substance, so the procedure is less of an ordeal.

The CAT scan is considerably easier on the patient. CAT stands for computerized axial tomography, a technique developed first in England before spreading rapidly to the United States.

The CAT scanner can take X-rays of parts of the body that do not form clear images on conventional X-rays. The scanner was used first on brains but now has been adapted to study other parts of the body. The technique has been particularly valuable in adding to the medical knowledge of back problems.

For a scan, the patient lies on a table with the part of the body to be studied within the machine. Beams of X-rays are passed through the body part and the transmitted signal is recorded on the other side. The beam and recorder are rotated around the body. All information is processed by a computer which, through a complex series of calculations, is able to construct a cross-dimensional image.

With a scan, physicians can spot disk problems and determine if any abnormalities in the shape or size of the vertebral canal may be causing problems. Some physicians also use the CAT scan to monitor the recovery of patients receiving conservative treatment.

Even this seemingly problem-free diagnostic test can cause controversy among doctors treating back problems.

One faction supports the use of CAT scans, arguing the scanner permits them to spot spinal anomalies missed in myelograms and surgery. It's claimed the CAT scan often uncovers facet joints pinching on nerves and other problems often overlooked.

Another segment of the medical community urges caution in the use of CAT scans. Physicians in this group declare the scans may reveal abnormalities in the spine and disk protrusions, but they may not be significant. These conditions may not be the cause of the patient's suffering, though their discovery might cause surgery to be performed needlessly.

That kind of controversy is common in the back problems world.

An article in *Medical World News*, entitled "Getting Aggressive About Conservative

Therapy for Back Pain," illustrates the diviseness among doctors on how back problems should be handled.

Some doctors quoted prescribe exercise for their patients. Others thought the role of exercise was overrated. Even the ones who agreed on exercise differed over what kind.

Similar controversy was expressed about other forms of treatment for back problems. One orthopedist favored spinal manipulation for lower-back pain; another gave up using it, considering it only a temporary solution.

Even the old stand-by treatment, bed rest, is a focus of disagreement. Some doctors feel bed rest is important while others say too much bed rest can further weaken the muscles and aggravate, instead of cure, the back problem.

The physicians can't be blamed for the diversity of their views. Despite the long history of back problems and the enormous financial cost, there have been no controlled studies to really define causes of back pain and to determine the effectiveness of various types of treatment. The kind of research needed for conventional double-blind studies seems impossible with the diffuse problems of the back patient. Back pain doesn't lend itself to absolute measures and research results would have to be based on subjective responses.

But there has been an explosion of knowledge in the last five years. And with each additional bit of information, the view of back problems becomes a little clearer.

The difficulty in diagnosing and treating back problems is hard both on the physician and the patient.

A physician at the Palo Alto Medical Foundation comments; "I think the back still goes begging. It's almost impossible, on the basis of an examination, to tell the patient, 'This is what you have and this is what it will take to get you better.'

"Most people leave the doctor's office uncertain what is going to happen. With pneumonia, you can say the patient will be well in two weeks. With a broken arm, you put it in a cast. But with backs, it's unclear."

The nebulous, indefinite quality of back problems frustrates many physicians who like to work with clearly defined diseases. These doctors feel it's a reflection of their ability as healers to have the same patient come back again and again with pain.

Other doctors are fascinated by the vagueness and uncertainty, and become like detectives, searching for the clue to the real cause of the problem.

The back patient, swamped in a maze of conflicting theories and frustrated by a backache that never goes away for good, is perhaps more prone than other patients to switch from one doctor to another. If their family doctor doesn't produce results, they may visit a chiropractor or try acupuncture. Eventually, the episode of back pain clears up.

In that sense, back problems are like colds. Except for the ones with definite medical causes, the average lower-back problem will normally get better, regardless of what the patient or doctor does.

FOUR:

MUSCLES OR DISKS?

A decade ago, the popular belief was that 80 percent of lower-back problems were caused by weak muscles.

A new theory has revolutionized that thinking. This philosophy holds that most back pain is caused by problems with intervertebral disks, the so-called "jelly doughnuts" separating vertebrae in the spinal column. This school reasons that protruding or slipped disks, pressing against nerves, are what give people the most trouble.

The pro-muscle group points to case histories of patients with weak muscles who recovered from back pain after developing stronger muscles. The pro-disk theorists note that many people with poor muscle tone have no back problems.

Some of the views of these two groups are exactly opposite.

Doctors subscribing to the muscle theory urge patients to do a "pelvic tilt" to take the curve out of the back.

The disk advocates advise just the opposite, recommending exercises to bend backward exaggerating the curve. Bending forward exercises are ordered in some cases, however. This is a part of the new philosophy — that all back cases are different and one prescription doesn't fit all patients.

Knowledge about back problems is still so imprecise, the final word isn't in yet on which faction is correct. Because of the complex nature of back problems, probably both sides have good points. The intelligent physician will pick and choose from both theories to find what seems most valid and most appropriate for the individual patient.

In an era when increasingly it has become important for health consumers to become involved in medical decisions, it's important for back patients to know what kinds of care are available to them. Then they can cooperate with their physicians in making intelligent choices about their health care.

An analysis of the muscles vs. disks theories is a requisite for the educated back patient.

THE MUSCLE SIDE

A key figure in arguing that weak muscles cause 80 percent of lower-back problems was Dr. Hans Kraus, former associate professor of physical medicine and rehabilitation at New York University and an internationally renowned specialist in the rehabilitation of athletic injuries and in back problems.

Kraus, in his book, *Backache, Stress and Tension: Cause, Prevention and Treatment,* writes, "Back pain and under-exercise are intimately related. Clinical studies show that more than 80 percent of all back pain cases are caused by under-exercise.

"If your muscles are weak and tense, lower-back pain can strike at any time," he warns. "Suddenly all the tension that has been building up in your system seems to focus across the lower back, just above the buttocks. In an instant, as you go to turn or twist, or to stoop or straighten up, muscles go into a wracking spasm. You cannot move. You are locked into position. You wonder what hit you. . . For a day or two the pain persists. Then slowly it ebbs. At last you manage to hobble out of bed. Then the pain seems to go away and you gingerly test your back. A week, a month, maybe two months later, the pain attacks again. This time it's worse. You wonder what's wrong, nothing seems to help.''

Kraus believes these patients can be helped, and if they had exercised properly, probably never would have needed help.

Kraus worked with Dr. Sonja Weber in the Posture Clinic of Columbia-Presbyterian Hospital in New York City, making detailed examinations of youngsters sent to the clinic with posture problems. Most of the patients were well and normal and were there only because of ''poor posture.''

Kraus and Weber noticed the children quickly learned how to stand in good posture, but slipped back into poor posture when no one was looking.

The doctors decided the poor posture was caused by a muscular inability to move properly. They devised a series of tests to measure muscle strength to help understand why the children slouched or were round-shouldered or sway-backed.

The original battery of 15 muscle tests was later reduced to six.

Weber and Kraus later participated in a special back clinic at Columbia-Presbyterian set up to find the cause for the ever-increasing number of back pain sufferers. Physicians at the hospital had made X-ray and laboratory tests of the patients, but in more than 80 percent of the cases, no abnormalities were found.

Kraus and Weber were supposed to study the muscular efficiency of that 80 percent who had no obvious reasons for their back problems. Six key tests were developed for the children in the posture clinic.

The six tests are:

1. Lie flat on your back on the floor with your hands clasped behind your neck and with your legs straight and touching. Keep your knees straight and lift your feet so that your heels are 10 inches above the floor. You pass the test if you can hold that position for 10 seconds.

This test shows if your hip flexors have sufficient strength.

2. Lie flat on the floor, again with your hands clasped behind your neck. Have someone hold down your legs by grasping the ankles, or hook your ankles under a heavy chair. Roll up to a sitting position. You pass if you can do one sit-up.

This test reveals whether or not your hip flexors and stomach muscles combined are strong enough to handle your body weight.

3. Again, lie flat on the floor with your hands behind your neck, only this time have

Kraus-Weber test #1

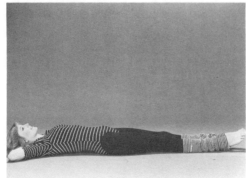

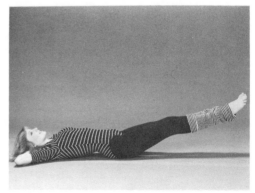

For Kraus-Weber test number one, lie flat on your back on the floor with your hands clasped behind your neck and with legs straight and touching.

Keep your knees straight and lift your feet so that your heels are 10 inches above the floor.

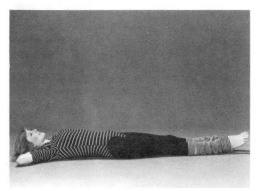

After holding legs 10 inches high for 10 seconds, slowly lower them back to floor.

Kraus-Weber test #2

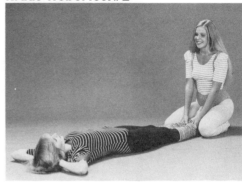

For Kraus-Weber number two, lie flat on floor, hands clasped behind neck. A helper grasps the ankles.

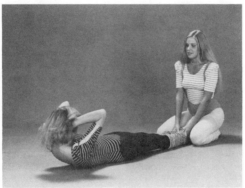

Start to roll up.

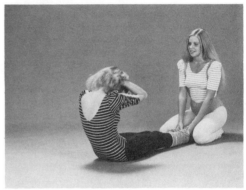

Rolling up almost vertical.

your knees flexed, heels close to the buttocks. Make sure your ankles are held down. Now roll up again to a sitting position.

This tests the strength of your stomach muscles.

4. Turn over on your stomach. Put a pillow under your abdomen, clasp your hands behind your neck and lie flat on the floor. Have your helper hold the lower half of your body steady by placing one hand in the small of the back and the other on the ankles. Now lift your trunk and hold it steady for 10 seconds.

This test reveals whether or not your back muscles are strong.

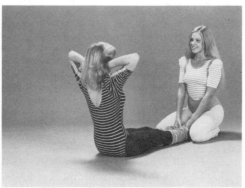

Rolled up to the sitting position—you pass test number two.

Kraus-Weber test #3

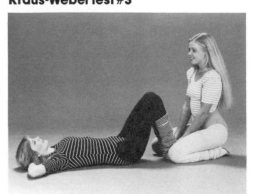

For Kraus-Weber test number three, again lie flat on the floor with hands behind the neck, but this time with knees flexed, heels close to the buttocks and ankles held down.

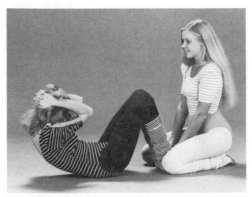

Start to roll up.

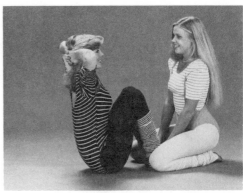

You pass if you can roll up to a sitting position.

Kraus-Weber test #4

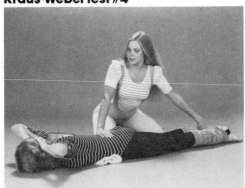

Lie on your stomach with a pillow under abdomen, clasping your hands behind neck. Helper holds body steady at the small of the back and ankles.

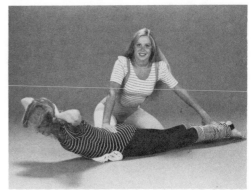

When ready, lift your trunk and hold steady for 10 seconds to see if your back muscles are strong.

Kraus-Weber test #5

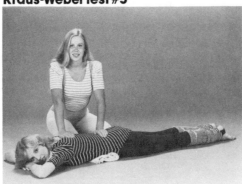

Kraus-Weber number five is also done on your stomach, folding your arms under your head and with a pillow under the abdomen.

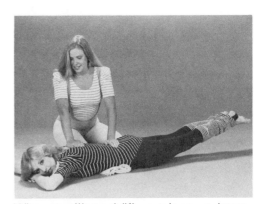

When positioned, lift your legs up, keeping the knees straight, and hold for 10 seconds.

5. Stay on your stomach, folding your arms under your head. Make sure the pillow is still under your abdomen. Have your helper hold your back steady with both hands. Now lift your legs up, being sure to keep your knees straight and hold the position for 10 seconds.

This tests the strength of your lower-back muscles.

6. For the last test, stand up straight, making sure your feet are together. Relax, lean over and touch the floor with your fingertips without bending your knees.

Kraus-Weber test #6

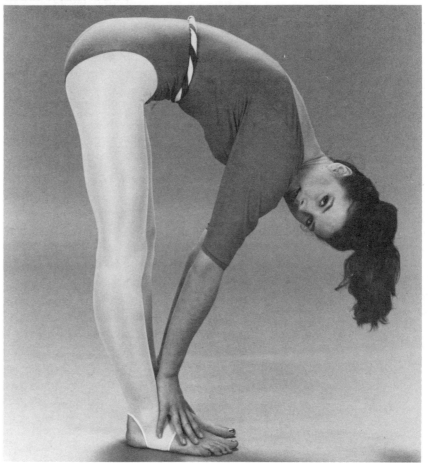

The sixth and final Kraus-Weber test involves standing up straight with your feet together, then relaxing and leaning over to touch the floor (modified to tops of feet, above) without bending the knees.

If you can pass this test, you have sufficient flexibility in your back muscles and hamstrings (the muscles in the back of your thighs). If you fail, it is because these muscles have become shortened and tense, not because your arms are too short or your legs are too long.

The Kraus-Weber tests are designed to determine only if the person meets minimum levels of muscular fitness. The two doctors believed that if a person failed even one of the tests, he was under par and needed help.

After testing the back patients at the Columbia-Presbyterian clinic, Kraus and Weber found they could determine not only whether patients were weak or tense, but also exactly what the deficiencies were.

Exercise works. Exercises were prescribed, with gratifying results. The patients who exercised faithfully were relieved of back pain in a few weeks or months. Those who did not exercise continued to suffer.

Kraus and Weber realized they not only had discovered an effective way of treating and relieving muscular back pain, but more importantly, had discovered a way of predicting potential back trouble.

They discovered the latter when they began giving the six tests to healthy people. Often a person who failed even one of the tests was a prime candidate for back trouble.

The initial reaction from the medical community to the Kraus-Weber theory that muscles were to blame in 80 percent of lower-back problems was unenthusiastic.

Kraus and Weber presented their findings to the annual meeting of the New York State Medical Society in 1954, receiving a cool reception. At that time, the idea that exercise was responsible for many ills was regarded as extremely radical. Kraus recalls that about that time a book was published, entitled "Exercise is Bosh."

The controversy spilled over into the press and was called to the attention of then President Dwight Eisenhower, who was concerned about studies showing the poor fitness levels of American children.

President Eisenhower later established the Council for Physical Fitness, the first step in what would become a new focus on exercise and physical fitness in the United States.

John F. Kennedy, who succeeded Eisenhower as president, also helped change the climate and encouraged the new emphasis on physical fitness. Kennedy was particularly interested in back problems because he himself suffered from back pain. Kraus served as his physician.

Kraus' experience convinced him a regular exercise program would benefit back patients. But he saw the program must include an element missing in other exercise programs. He realized stress and tension were important factors in creating back problems, so he included relaxation training in his program.

After following a series of patients for two to eight years, Kraus discovered symptoms of the patients diminished as they increased muscle strength and flexibility.

There was a problem, however. The number of back patients who might benefit from exercise programs was too large to be handled either in private medical practices or in hospital clinics.

He sought a way to make exercise programs available to large numbers of people.

YMCA program. In the 1970s, a pilot program was started at several New York City YMCAs. Physical educators there were trained to teach a program that included simple relaxation training, limbering and warm-up exercises and abdominal strengthening routines. By reversing the sequence of exercises, the routine ended with cool-off exercises and finally relaxation again.

After a feasibility study, 300 physical fitness educators were trained across the country by Kraus and by the program's national consultant, Alexander Melleby.

The program was called "The Y's Way to a Healthy Back." In March, 1976, it was established as a national program with the six-week course offered at YMCAs across the nation.

In the first year of the program, 400 people enrolled. By now almost every one of the nearly 2000 YMCAs in the country offer the program. More than 200,000 people have completed the course.

A survey of the results showed that about 65 percent of the back patients completing the course reported they were either in excellent condition (all pain had disappeared and they could do everything) or in good condition (much less pain and able to do most things).

The program produced results at minimal cost, too, always important with the spiraling costs of health care.

Among the exercises included in the Y's Way to a Healthy Back is this one for relaxation:

• Lie on the floor, flexing the knees. Slowly draw one knee and then the other as close to the chest as comfortable.

Two stretching exercises from the program are the Pectoral Stretch and the Cat Back.

• For the Pectoral Stretch, participants kneel, place their hands and forearms on the floor and gradually slide forward on their arms, keeping back and head straight.

YMCA relaxation exercise

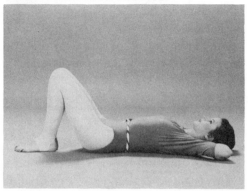

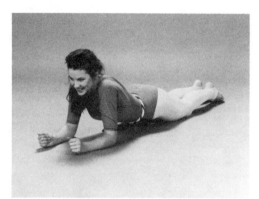

For the YMCA's Relaxation Exercise, lie on the floor, flexing the knees.

Then draw one knee as close to the chest as comfortable, lower and draw the other knee up.

YMCA pectoral stretch

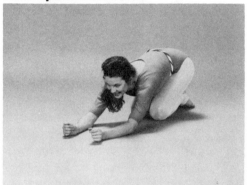

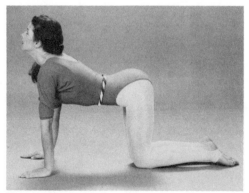

For the YMCA's Pectoral Stretch, first kneel and place your hands and fore-arms on the floor.

Then gradually slide forward on your arms, keeping back and head straight.

YMCA cat back

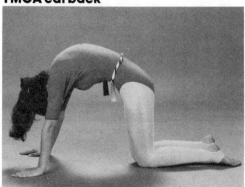

In the YMCA's Cat Back, arch your back like a cat while dropping your head.

Then alternate by reversing the arch, bringing your head up.

• In the Cat Back, participants positioned on their hands and knees alternately arch their backs like a cat, dropping their heads at the same time. They then reverse the arch, bringing their heads up. They inhale on the arch, exhale on the sway.

The idea that exercise is good for everybody and may be especially helpful for back patients is well-established now. We live in an exercising society and patients have come to expect their doctors to give them exercises for their back problems.

Even advocates of the disk theory of back problems accept the fact that the spine works with surrounding muscle groups. Strong abdominal muscles help to bear the weight of the body. Leg muscles should be strong enough for a person to use his legs in lifting. And it's important to stretch the hamstring muscles that move the hips and knees and to stretch the heel cords.

A sampling of the exercises prescribed for back patients at the Palo Alto Medical Foundation follows:

1. Low back warm-up and coordination exercise. Assume the hand knee position on the floor. Arch back as far as possible, then slowly relax and allow a full low back curve. Raise opposite arm and leg at the same time. Repeat on the opposite side. Repeat each exercise at least 10 times.

2. Single knee to chest. Start in the hook lying position: Lie flat on your back with your knees bent and feet on the floor. Using your hands, pull one knee to your chest. Return to the starting position. Repeat on the opposite side. Use the rhythm of "pressure on, pressure off." Repeat on each side.

Lower-back warmup

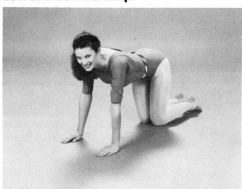

For the Palo Alto Medical Foundation's Lower-Back Warmup and Coordination Exercise, assume the hand knee position on the floor.

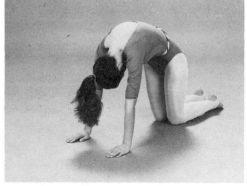

Then arch the back as far as possible.

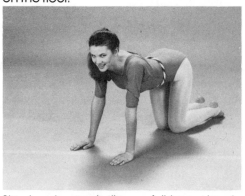

Slowly relax and allow a full lower-back curve.

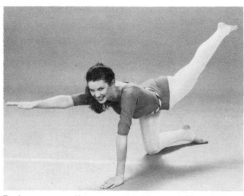

Raise opposite arm and leg at the same time.

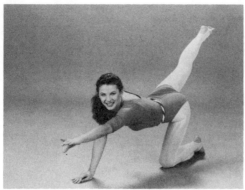

Repeat, raising arm and leg on the other side.

Single knee to chest

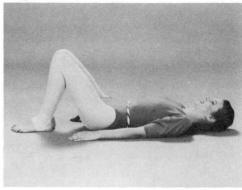

Start in the hook lying position for the Single Knee to Chest Exercise. Lie flat on your back on the floor with your knees bent and feet on the floor.

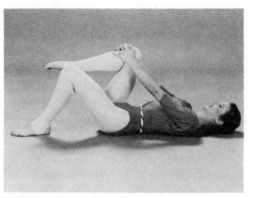

Using your hands, pull one knee up....

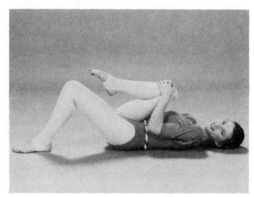

...until the knee is pulled up to your chest. Then repeat on the opposite side.

3. Double knee to chest. Start in the hook lying position: Lie flat on your back with your knees bent and your feet on the floor. Using your hands, pull both knees to your chest. Return to the starting position. Use the rhythm of "pressure on, pressure off."

4. Partial sit-ups. (Strong abdominal muscles are essential to good body mechanics, posture and compression during heavy lifting, Palo Alto Medical Foundation doctors explain. Full sit-ups are often taught for strengthening these muscles. However, studies have shown that the strongest abdominal contraction comes during the initial part of the sit-up and that the leg and hip muscles pull the trunk into a full sit-up.)

(Studies also demonstrate a high intra-joint pressure during a full sit-up. In order to reduce the strain on the lower back and strengthen the abdominals effectively, a partial sit-up is all that is required.)

In the beginning of your exercise program, do a partial sit-up by crossing your arms over your chest and lifting your head and shoulders (as far as your shoulder blades) off the floor and hold for 15 seconds. Repeat three times. After a week, begin to increase the length of time the exercise is held and the number of repetitions.

5. Hamstring stretch. Tight hamstrings may interfere with back flexibility. To stretch this muscle group, place one foot on a chair and place both hands on the upper thigh for support. Lower your body toward the knee, keeping your knees straight and supporting your body weight with your hands on your thigh until a good stretch is felt under the

Double knee to chest

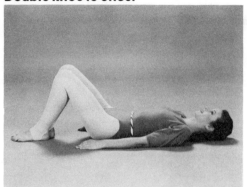

For the Palo Alto Medical Foundation's Double Knee to Chest, also start by lying on your back with knees bent and feet on the floor.

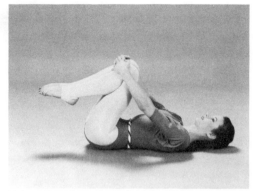

Using your hands, pull up both knees . . .

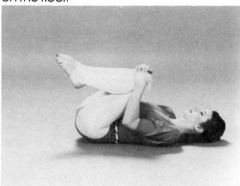

. . . until the knees are pulled up to your chest. Then return to starting position.

Partial sit-ups

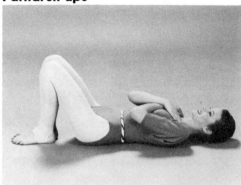

For strengthening the abdominal muscles, the Palo Alto Medical Foundation's Partial Situps begin lying flat on your back with knees bent and arms crossed over your chest.

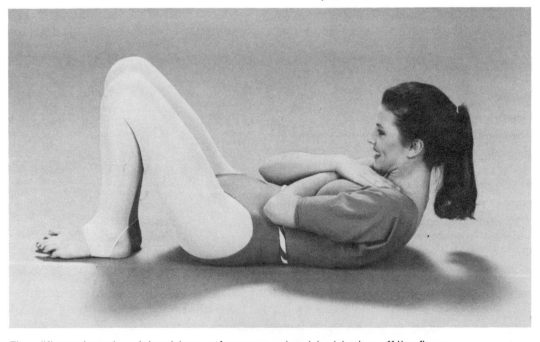

Then lift your head and shoulders, as far as your shoulder blades, off the floor.

Heel cord stretch

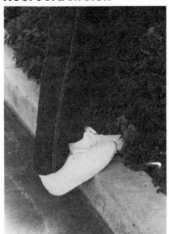

Hamstring stretch

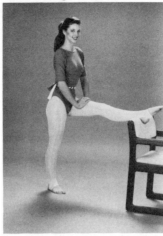

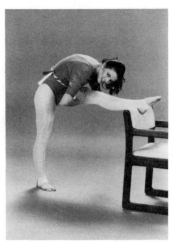

To do Heel Cord Stretch, allow one heel to hang off a step while keeping the knee straight. Hold long enough to follow the rhythm: "pressure on, pressure off."

For the Hamstring Stretch, place one foot on a chair and both hands on upper thigh.

Lower body toward knee, keeping knees straight, supporting weight with hands on thigh.

thighs and knee. Be sure that the stretch is felt equally on each side of the knee. Use the rhythm of "pressure on, pressure off." Repeat at least twice a day, five to 10 times on each leg. For a stronger stretch, use a higher chair or table.

6. Heel cord stretch. Stand on a step and keep your knee straight. Allow one heel to hang off the end of the step. Use something for balance. Hold stretch only long enough to follow the rhythm of "pressure on, pressure off." Then repeat on the other side.

Or stand approximately four feet away from a wall. Place hands shoulder high and a shoulder width apart. Keeping one leg straight, lean until you feel a good stretch in your calf. Repeat with other leg using the rhythm of "pressure on, pressure off."

Exercises only work when the back patient does them. Too often a person will follow his prescribed exercise routine faithfully as long as his back is acting up or the memory of the backache is still fresh in his mind.

Then, he feels better and the exercises don't seem as important. In our hurried existence, there is never enough time, and it's hard to find 10 to 15 minutes daily to exercise.

It's largely a matter of self-discipline. People can schedule in their lives whatever they feel is important. Frequently, they don't realize exercise is that important until after their second or third bout with back pain.

By then even the most reluctant exerciser is usually a convert.

THE DISK SIDE

Traditionally, physical therapists have treated patients with lower-back problems by cautioning them to keep their backs straight to decrease the lower lumbar curve.

Patients were taught the pelvic tilt as a maneuver to protect the lower back. They were told to tuck their buttocks under, flattening the spine and putting the stomach in a better position to support and protect the back.

In recent years there's been a complete turnaround in that thinking. Patients now are advised to keep the natural curve in the lower back at all times, particularly when sitting.

As with all other theories in back care, this one isn't accepted universally. But it is a theory that is rapidly gaining acceptance and is used at many medical institutions throughout the world.

The Palo Alto Medical Foundation's physical therapy department adopted the new ideas about three years ago. Kaiser Permanente Medical Center in California, a health maintenance organization, also pioneered the new theory.

Two leading doctors who argue that disks and nerves are the cause of most back problems are James Cyriax and Robin McKenzie.

Cyriax, a world authority on the slipped disk, is honorary consulting physician in orthopedic medicine at St. Thomas's Hospital, London, and visiting professor in orthopedic medicine at Rochester University Medical Center in New York.

McKenzie, a native of New Zealand, was a physical therapist in private practice in Wellington in 1953, when he developed a strong interest in back problems.

(Cyriax and McKenzie's nationalities reflect the fact, acknowledged by most American doctors, that Britain and the commonwealth nations are ahead of the United States in back care.)

McKenzie's interest was aroused after he treated sheep shearers, who often worked 10 hours a day in a bent-over position. He would see 20 to 30-year-old men with 80-year-old backs.

Although both doctors agreed that disk lesions were largely at fault in back problems, each has his own ideas of the best way to treat them. Cyriax favors use of manipulation of the spine, while McKenzie advocates correct posture and body mechanics.

In contrast to followers of the "muscle school," Cyriax declares emphatically, "Disk trouble is all but universal."

In his book, "The Slipped Disk," he writes, "Few people reach middle age without suffering at one time or another with a crick in the neck, pain in one shoulder blade, neuritis in the arm, pain at the back of the chest perhaps radiating around to the ribs in front, backache, lumbago, sacroiliac strain or sciatica . . . These symptoms are commonly occurring with different types of slipped disks at different levels around the spinal column."

Although Cyriax uses the term "slipped disk," he notes that it is inaccurate, commenting, "The whole disk does not slip out like a penny from a slot; indeed, as long as it is structurally sound, it cannot move. It is only when a crack has developed as the result of injury or of years of wear and tear, and has led to the formation of a loose piece, that this small fragment can shift and cause so much recurrent trouble."

Cyriax bases his ideas on his understanding of how the spinal column functions, and the role of the two curves in the spine. In his view, the curves were developed to mitigate the bad effects of compression on the spinal disks. The two curves produce a tilt on the joint surfaces at the weakest levels that exerts a forward pressure on the disk.

As long as the curves are maintained, the squashy gel-like disk is pushed forward, away from the dura mater, the membrane covering the spinal cord and the nerve roots. This protective feature means less danger of a protruding disk pressing against nerves and causing back pain.

Cyriax goes against many conventional ideas in urging that postural exercises designed to eliminate the normal spinal curve, such as the pelvic tilt, should be discredited.

He urges abandoning any exercise that involves bending down and touching the toes, rejecting the "fetish" that no one is fit unless he can bend and touch his toes. Rather, he declares, the ability is dependent on the length of the person's hamstring muscles at the back of the thigh, and long ones are no better than short ones.

Cyriax is one of the back experts who believe that the current increase in disk problems, at a time when the amount of heavy labor people do has lessened, is caused by the amount of sitting we do.

"Whereas we used to walk everywhere, stood in the presence of our betters and sat very upright at meals, keeping the back hollow,' " he writes, "we now slouch in arm-chairs, cars and airplanes, the back rounded for long periods of time.

"As a result the disk is subjected to continuous centrifugal pressure at the very time when the back is held convex. This posture entails the very tilt on the joint surfaces that forces the disk backwards towards the sensitive nervous tissue. This is the first time in history that man has spent so much time sitting — the worst posture to adopt from the point of view of the disk."

Cyriax also has an explanation of why disk problems — and consequently back problems — recur. He points out that the outer ring of the disk surrounding the soft nucleus is cartilage, the only tissue in the body not containing blood.

If a bone breaks or the skin is cut, healing takes place. But that can't happen with the annulus fibrosus, the ring surrounding the disk nucleus. Once split, the edges can never join together. The same kind of tear in cartilage occurs in a knee of a football player. A torn piece stays loose, and if it causes annoynance, it has to be removed.

McKenzie differs with Cyriax on this point. He believes scar tissue can form over the split.

Cyriax says if a fragment of a disk comes loose, as in a slipped or ruptured disk, the loose piece may slip back into position by itself. It may be reduced by manipulation or traction or it may slowly edge back into position during relief from compression, as when the sufferer rests in bed. But the loose fragment always stays free and may slip out of place again.

SUSCEPTIBILITY TO PAIN

McKenzie believes there are three factors that increase susceptibility to lower-back pain.

The sitting posture. A good sitting posture maintains the normal curves of the spine. Poor posture reduces or accentuates the normal curves and stretches the ligaments of the spine, causing pain.

Loss of lumbar extension. This is the ability to bend backwards. He quotes studies that show from 75 to 86 percent of patients with lower-back pain had a loss of extension, influencing posture in sitting, standing and walking.

Frequency of flexion. The lifestyle of Western cultures calls for much bending over and stooping at home and at work, leading to a loss of ability to extend the spine. (Key words in McKenzie's philosophy are flexion and extension. Flexion refers to the motion of bending forward or stooping, and extension to the motion of bending the back backward.)

A trivial movement or lifting may cause back pain but McKenzie believes the real cause is repeated movements in daily life that are bad for the back.

BACK PROBLEM SYNDROMES

McKenzie, who confines his attention only to mechanical causes of back pain, classifies back problems into three syndromes.

The postural syndrome. It results from postural stresses, causes intermittent pain brought on by a particular position or posture.

The dysfunction syndrome. Changes in the soft tissues of the back that lead to an adaptive shortening, creating a consequent restriction in movement. It is characterized by intermittent pain and a partial loss of movement.

The derangement syndrome. Alterations in the fluid nucleus within the disk and possibly in the surrounding annulus, causing a change in the position of the disk between the two vertebrae.

Various forms and degrees of derangement are possible; each presents different symptoms and requires different treatments.

Agreeing with Cyriax on the prominence of disk problems, McKenzie asserts that as many as 95 percent of the patients he sees have back problems caused by disks.

CORRECTING POSTURE

To correct pain caused by the postural syndrome, he believes only a correction of posture is needed.

He teaches patients how to sit properly, maintaining the curve — or lordosis — in the lower back either by using their own muscles or by using a lumbar support. After 10 days, he expects postural pain will be gone.

McKenzie's theory goes against much accepted practice in the United States, where the aim has been to eliminate the curve in the back and where flexion has been considered beneficial and extension undesirable.

He also rejects what he terms a "popular misconception" that the posture can be corrected by strengthening the muscles of the spine. He emphasizes that strengthening the muscles has no effect on posture and only by maintaining correct posture can back pain be alleviated.

To treat dysfunction, McKenzie prescribes movements that produce pain on the theory that the movement gradually will stretch the soft tissues of the back, correcting the mechanical problems.

Exercises are prescribed according to the nature of the patient's limitations. The most common problem is restriction of the ability to bend backwards. To correct it, he has patients do press-ups and other exercises to extend the back. For the patient who has trouble bending forward, McKenzie prescribes the same type of forward bending (flexion) exercises often given to all types of back patients in the United States.

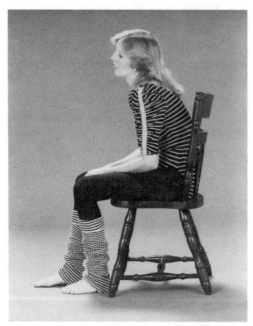

Poor posture when sitting reduces or accentuates the normal curves in the spine, stretching the ligaments and causing pain.

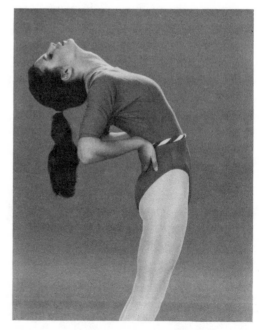

Many back patients lose their ability to bend backwards, adversely affecting their posture while sitting, standing and walking.

Patients are told to bend to the point of pain because they must stretch the ligaments and muscles.

For the derangement syndromes where disks are involved, McKenzie believes disturbance of the intervertebral disk is responsible for producing symptoms.

He's been convinced by his experience that the problems occur because of the hydrostatic properties of the disk. He feels there is ample evidence that movements of the spinal column affect the position of the jelly-like nucleus of the disk. Pressure of bending can push the substance of the disk either forward, backward or sideways, depending on the motion of the spine.

Patients with derangement syndrome are commonly between 20 and 55 years of age. From that time on, disk problems reduce gradually as degenerative processes develop.

McKenzie also believes men are affected more often by disk problems than are women.

Derangement syndrome is marked by the recurrent nature of the pain. It's estimated as many as 60 to 90 percent of these patients will have recurring bouts with pain.

While patients with postural or dysfunctional problems have intermittent pain, the derangement syndrome causes constant pain. And while sitting is the most common aggravating factor for all lower-back pain patients, only with disk problems does the pain increase when rising from a sitting position.

In the early acute stages of derangement, McKenzie insists only that the patient maintain the lower-back curve (lordosis). Usually a patient understands the risks of bending and stooping and avoids those movements. But often he doesn't realize the hidden dangers of sitting in a slouched position.

McKenzie also may use mobilization or manipulation techniques in treating these patients.

He assumes that when the patient can bend backward without pain, the derangement has been reduced. At that point, he prescribes flexion exercises. Patients are allowed to resume most of their activities, provided they follow McKenzie's advice on prevention tactics.

For severe disk problems accompanied by sciatica (a nerve involvement), McKenzie doesn't feel mechanical therapy is sufficient. He notes continous traction in bed may produce good results; otherwise, surgery may be needed.

McKenzie's philosophy of treatment is strongly endorsed by Dr. Arthur H. White, director of St. Mary's Spine Center and founder of the California Back School in San Francisco, Calif. White reports 20 percent of his patients are more responsive to McKenzie's methods than to any of the methods used in the past. Because White sees back patients with chronic problems, he believes these techniques would help 50 to 80 percent of the patients seen in early stages of back problems.

SELF-HELP BACK CARE

McKenzie, an enthusiast of self-help back care, believes people can treat their own back problems by following a few simple rules.

Among them are:

Sit properly. Maintain the curve in your lower back, perhaps through the help of a lumbar supportive roll.

Interrupt prolonged sitting. Research shows that even when a person sits correctly, the pressure on the disk is increased while sitting and prolonged pressure may cause some distortion in the joints containing the disks.

No bending. Keep to a minimum working in a stooped or bent over position. If it is necessary, then counteract the adverse effects by doing an exercise that's a McKenzie standard: backward bending while standing. He feels that backward bending done before pain starts will usually prevent significant lower-back pain.

Don't relax. After vigorous activity, don't slouch down in an easy chair. Thoroughly exercised joints in the lower-back can distort easily if put in that position. Instead, do some backward bending, or if you do sit down to rest, sit in a straight chair in an upright position.

Lift correctly. Always maintain the hollow in the lower back. Bend your knees and hold the load close to you.

Flatten the back. After prolonged standing, flatten the back when the lower-back curve may hang in an extreme curved position, adopt the pelvic tilt position and flatten the curve by pulling on the stomach muscles and tightening the buttock muscles.

Sleep on a firm mattress. If you have pain while lying down, sleep on a hard surface. If that doesn't bring relief, use a supportive roll to fill the natural hollow in the body between pelvis and rib cage when lying on your side or beneath the lower back if lying on your back.

McKenzie also warns of high-risk situations: traveling long distances by auto, removing heavy objects from the trunk of your car immediately after driving, traveling by plane, working in a stooped position especially during the first hours of the day, and coughing and sneezing when you are bent forward or sitting.

His advice for the person with a cold and lower-back problems is: "You must try to stand up and bend backwards while coughing or sneezing. At least lean back and make the best lordosis (excessive arching) you can."

Otherwise, a cough or sneeze can cause a sudden attack of lower-back pain or aggravate an existing problem.

McKenzie's self-treatment plan also includes a simple exercise routine, with most of the movements designed to increase the curve in the lower back.

THE PROBLEM OF TOO-STRONG MUSCLES

Weak muscles may lead to back problems, but even people with strong muscles may experience back difficulties.

Usually in these cases it's a question of someone overdoing or overexerting his back. Or it may be a misuse of the body so that even with strong muscles, a back problem develops. Even a college athlete, an avid runner, a teen-age swimming star or a professional football player may be plagued by back problems.

Just because a person has good muscles in his arms and legs doesn't mean the back muscles are strong. And many athletic people push their backs too far. A runner may get caught up in the competition with himself to add more and more miles to his weekly stint. He may end up with a back problem if he doesn't carry himself properly.

Gymnasts, too, are examples of strong athletes who can develop back problems because of the extreme contortions they put their spine through. This risk is not serious for young gymnasts because their spines are not well developed, but they still may do structural damage to their backs.

Swimming usually is considered a safe activity for the average person, but it can be hazardous if you concentrate too much on one thing. A research study showed teen-age swimmers developed back problems after excessive practice of the butterfly stroke. The other styles of swimming caused no problems.

Professional athletes have their share of back problems too. However, pros are in an enviable position for treatment. Their body's health means their livelihood, and trainers and physical therapists are available to them immediately to deal with developing back problems.

FIVE:

TREATMENTS BEYOND EXERCISE

Exercise isn't the only prescription physicians have for back patients and, in fact, exercise normally comes later, after the acute bout of pain is under control.

Medications don't play a large part in the treatment of generalized back problems caused by weak muscles, tension or disk problems. Aspirin, pain killers, nonsteroidal anti-inflammatory drugs, muscle relaxants, perhaps anti-depressants, are used. They relieve symptoms and make the patient feel better, but don't cure the disease.

This is one reason back problems can be so frustrating to the patient and doctor alike. It's not possible to write a prescription for antibiotics and know the patient will recover before all the pills are taken. Chemotherapy and radiation, mainstays in treating cancer, are of no use in treating back problems where no malignancies are present, even though the pain may be almost as severe.

Among the possible treatments a physician may prescribe are these:

BED REST

Bed rest has been the classic prescription for back patients throughout history. Surprisingly, it's still considered an effective way to alleviate lower-back problems.

Lying horizontally takes the pressure off the spine and allows the conditions that brought the acute flare-up of pain to ease off. For pain caused by a disk problem, lying down lowers the intradiscal pressure. At the same time, it can allow inflammation around a nerve root to calm down.

The prescribing of hospital bed rest has declined a bit, especially since room rates have zoomed, making a hospital stay exorbitantly expensive. Formerly, a patient might be hospitalized for several weeks or a month or more, with strict orders to stay absolutely quiet, not even getting up to go to the bathroom.

Today, it's more likely the patient will rest at home in his own bed. And the rules may be more lenient. He will be allowed up for trips to the bathroom and even perhaps for meals. It's important the bed be suitable — firm and flat — and that the patient lie in the proper position.

Amazingly often, a few days in bed will clear up even severe lower-back pain and sciatica, the pain in the leg caused by pressure on the sciatic nerve. Normally, bed rest continues until the pain has gone away. Even afterward, the patient may be advised to take daily periods of rest, especially if the back problem is chronic.

Even bed rest patients aren't allowed to avoid exercises. To counteract the weakening of muscles that occurs during long periods of lying down, a physician may prescribe simple exercises to do in bed to maintain muscle tone. These could include tightening the abdominal muscles and squeezing the buttocks together, or, if not too painful, straight leg raising.

INJECTIONS

Not all medications need be taken by mouth and injections play a role in the treatment of back problems. However, here it is usually not the substance injected that's important but the process of injecting.

43

Injections most often are used to relieve the pain caused by trigger points, hard nodules that form in the back, perhaps in reaction to the stress of severe muscle spasms. Pressing on a trigger point elicits pain.

A doctor may inject a substance such as lidocaine, needling the trigger point from different angles. The lidocaine, an anesthetic, dulls the immediate pain of the injection. It is believed the cure comes from the puncturing of the trigger point and the fluid pressure the injection creates.

Injections also may be used for facet joint nerve blocks. Because pain can be caused by damage to the tiny facet joints between the vertebrae, the theory is that blocking the nerves coming from the joints would cut off the pain.

Rather than prescribing large doses of cortisone to help relieve inflammation around the facet joints, the physician may choose to inject a smaller amount of the medication instead. It's a tricky process because the injection must be placed in exactly the right spot.

If there appears to be an inflammation of the nerve roots, then an epidural injection may be performed: An anesthetic and cortisone are injected into the vertebral canal.

Injections do have one advantage. They have a tremendous placebo effect and may make the patient feel better even if nothing actually has changed. For the back patient that may not matter as much as the gratifying feeling that at least his doctor is doing something for him.

CORSETS

Corsets and braces are another form of traditional treatment. They are used to restrict motion of the lower back, to give abdominal support and to help the body maintain correct posture.

Sometimes corsets are used when patients won't or can't do exercises that would help their own muscles do the job taken over by an artificial support. The corsets also help serve as a restraint to remind the patient he can't bend and move as easily as he could before back pain started.

Ideally, corsets should be worn for a relatively short time so that muscles don't become dependent on the support and the corset becomes a crutch.

Sometimes workers such as garbage collectors may wear strong girdles while they work. The corsets appear to help the workers carry heavy loads with less strain on their back.

TRACTION

Hippocrates, the ancient Greek physician who became known as the father of medicine, may have been the first to develop the idea of traction for back patients. The beginning is so far back in history no one knows for sure.

The treatment has been used through the centuries, although there is no conclusive evidence of effectiveness.

The principle today is about the same as in Hippocrates' time. It is based on the fact that the spine, like an accordion, can be compressed and stretched. The idea of traction is literally to stretch the spine to counteract the shortening of the spine that results from the pressure of standing or sitting. Traction presumably alleviates the problem by opening up the space between vertebrae.

A do-it-yourself form of traction is possible. A person can stand against a door with his hands hooked over the upper edge. Gradually relax and bend the knees until the feet are lifted off the floor. It should be done slowly and carefully, gradually transferring weight to the feet before the hands tire.

Complicated hospital traction systems are available, although again fewer patients are hospitalized for traction than in the past. Physical therapists also use traction for patients. Most often, the patient will be placed in traction for only short periods.

Another form of traction, called "gravity lumbar traction," was first developed in the 1960s. It's a hanging traction device by which the patient hangs upside down over an upper thigh support, with hips bent at right angles.

In another form of gravity traction, patients are strapped to a tilting bed and rotated to an almost standing position.

Also currently getting attention are the gravity boots, a medieval-type traction system that allows the person to literally hang by his heels. There are various types called gravity guiding systems or gravity boots. The system was developed by Dr. Robert Martin of southern California, who found gravity boots helped relieve back pain in many of his patients.

The idea has caught on and users range from singer Wayne Newton to members of the U.S. Olympic weightlifting team. In using the system, a person fastens the boots on while in an upright position, then swings up so he is hanging upside down. It's possible to do exercises while in that position.

Despite glowing reports from some users, there are words of caution too. The system may be dangerous for persons with detached retinas, high blood pressure or some degenerative back problems. Some physicians also warn that it can be dangerous getting in and out of the system.

MANIPULATION

Manipulation, like traction, is a treatment that has been used through the centuries, but there still is no scientific data on how it works or if it does indeed work.

But it has been used successfully with many patients and if other modes of treatment fail, manipulation may be suggested. It will more commonly be prescribed by an osteopath or chiropractor than by an M.D.

Webster's dictionary defines manipulation as a "handling or being handled, especially skillful handling or operation," and that definition serves for the procedure as used for back problems.

In early times it was thought pain occurred because bones were out of alignment and could be manipulated back into line.

Generally, in manipulation, a particular segment of the spine is put through a range of motion, either slowly and gently or rapidly with more force. A manipulation always should be done by someone with a good knowledge of anatomy. Slow motions are generally safer than rapid ones. Manipulation can be done either painfully or without pain, and sometimes is done while the patient is under traction or is anesthetized.

The manipulations may realign the vertebrae and facet joints to relieve pain, or change the position of the disk nucleus, relieving pressure on a nerve. Possibly, too, the manipulation may change the position of the nerve roots in relation to the rest of the spine. Again, it's one of the mysteries that abound in the treatment of back problems.

When it works, it seems to do so almost immediately. Most experts feel that if manipulation doesn't succeed in two or three tries, it should be dropped as a treatment.

What Treatment Works Best?

Physicians are becoming increasingly aware that back patients use an enormous volume of medical services. Only routine examinations, postoperative checkups and upper respiratory tract symptoms top back problems as causes for office visits to doctors.

Most doctors agree that conservative treatment should be tried. Yet they are sensitive to the fact there is little scientific evidence to support the effectiveness of whichever therapy they might choose.

Should the patient have bed rest, traction, manipulation? Nothing points to an absolute answer. Rather, the doctor relies on personal biases and subjective feelings on what might be best for the patient.

The difficulty of defining the effectiveness of these different therapies was discovered by Dr. Richard A. Deyo, of the division of general internal medicine, Department of Medicine, at the University of Texas Health Science Center in San Antonio.

Deyo, reporting in the *Journal of the American Medical Association* on his efforts to research the effectiveness of the different therapies noted that most physicians agree the conservative treatments should be tried.

The large number of choices, he indicated, attest to the absence of a clearly superior method.

"Conflicting claims exist for nearly all of these," he wrote. "It is important to ascertain the efficacy of the treatments since many entail expense, work loss and risk of side effects."

Deyo found it was easier to say that than to do it.

He reviewed scientific literature on the different treatments, examining how the research was conducted, how patients were followed up and what the conclusions were. He found design flaws in many of the research projects and discovered little attention was paid to actually measuring a patient's compliance with the treatment in question.

Even discounting those basic problems, the research failed to present any conclusive results.

A study of three most commonly recommended exercise regimens showed no one set to have an advantage over the other two, or over corsets, traction or manipulation.

Bed rest has long been a mainstay of conservative treatment because patients often report symptomatic relief and the horizontal position reduces intradiscal pressure, Deyo noted. For these reasons, its value for patients with a herniated disk isn't disputed.

Whether bed rest is beneficial to patients without typical disk symptoms remains uncertain. There is no measure available on the optimal length of time a patient should remain in bed.

Only one study compared bed rest with continued activity. This study involved military recruits whose compliance could be enforced. Recruits assigned to bed rest experienced less pain and returned to full duty sooner than those required to remain ambulatory.

But this study was not the preferred double-blind model where the investigator doesn't know which therapy is being given to a patient — allowing for a possibility of investigator bias. Any studies comparing different durations of bed rest or analyzing type of patients for bed rest, are lacking. Deyo reported spinal manipulation remains controversial, partly because in the United States it is often equated with the practice of chiropractic.

In Great Britain and the commonwealth nations, spinal manipulation by physicians and physical therapists is more common and several clinical trials have been conducted.

Possible benefits of manipulation include reduction of a bulging disk caused by tightening of the ligaments, freeing of adhesions around a slipped disk, and mechanical stimulation of certain large nerve fibers which may inhibit the transmission of pain impulses.

However, different manipulation techniques were used in each study, and some of the patients receiving manipulations also were receiving traction at the same time. Deyo concluded the two best studies suggested some immediate benefit from manipulation, but no long-term benefits.

"Given the ubiquity of lower-back pain, its importance to society and its impact on the delivery of medical services, both the quantity and quality of therapeutic research in this area are disappointing," he concluded.

SURGERY

The whole picture of back care changed dramatically in 1934 when two Boston surgeons, W.G. Mixter and J.S. Barr, performed the first operation that was to be called a laminectomy.

The two doctors had been treating a young male patient for what they thought might be a tumor on the spine. During surgery, however, they found a protrusion at the back of the intervertebral disk pressing on a nerve root. They removed the protrusion and the patient was cured.

This success convinced the orthopedic surgeons that protrusions of the disks were a major cause of back problems. If so, it followed that surgical treatment was in order.

This idea quickly became popular, especially in view of the frustrating picture of back care. When it was thought back problems were caused by wear and tear on the spine, nothing could be done. Now, suddenly, a miraculous cure opened up.

It quickly led to what Dr. Oakley Hewitt, an orthopedic surgeon at the Palo Alto Medical Foundation, calls the "Dynasty of the Disks." From 1934 until the 1960s, disks were held responsible for almost all back problems.

It led to a wave of surgery. Many patients were having two or three laminectomies, but unfortunately, many patients ended up surgical cripples.

The fear that surgery is inevitable for back problems is a carryover from the dynasty of the disks. Patients have friends or family members who had poor results and often they will open a talk with their doctor by declaring emphatically, "No surgery for me. I'll do anything to avoid the knife."

However, laminectomies properly done are still considered a valid treatment for the patients diagnosed carefully with back problems amenable to surgery. Nearly 200,000 laminectomies are performed each year in the United States, a figure many doctors think is still too high.

The conservative doctor will do a laminectomy only as a last resort after other less traumatic treatments have failed to produce results. For the operation, the patient is placed face down on the operating table. An incision is made in the middle of the back in the area of the ruptured disk. The surgeon strips away the ligaments to enlarge the space to work, and then moves the spinal cord out of the way.

One surgeon, stressing the delicacy of this maneuver, explains the spinal cord is moved "very carefully." Then the fragment of the disk causing the back pain is excised.

Sometimes a follow-up operation, called a spinal fusion, is done. The disk between two vertebrae is removed and the vertebrae are fused together. Bone chips, usually taken from the pelvis, are laid between the adjoining vertebrae, becoming a permanent bond with the bone. That section of the spine becomes rigid. Spinal fusions used to be more popular. Now they are rarely done.

While laminectomies are accepted treatment, there is always a reluctance by the conscientous surgeon to operate unless absolutely necessary.

"With a back patient, one bite of the apple is all you get," Hewitt emphasizes. "After the first surgery, if it doesn't work, everything else you can do is a compromise."

CHYMOPAPAIN

Thanks to the papaya, and to a researcher who discovered the special properties of an enzyme taken from this tropical fruit, back patients now can choose a non-surgical treatment for disk problems.

It promises to be a boon to the one percent of all adult Americans who may suffer at some time in their lives from a herniated or slipped disk.

The papain enzyme (chymopapain) was first isolated in 1941, but its unique property was not discovered until 1956. The discovery was made by Dr. Lewis Thomas, an author and medical commentator who at that time was a pathologist at New York University-Bellevue Medical Center.

He discovered that when the substance was injected into the tall, rigid ears of rabbits, it caused the ears to collapse. It does so by dissolving the cartilage that holds the rabbit's ears upright. It is this quality that makes chymopapain work when injected into a herniated disk, dissolving the disk material (a form of cartilage) and relieving the pressure that causes pain.

As with most medical advances, it was a long time — seven years in this case — before this knowledge was used for a practical application. Dr. Lyman Smith, an Illinois orthopedic surgeon, developed chemonucleolysis, a technique in which chymopapain is injected into the herniated lumbar intervertebral disk that is causing back pain.

Clinical trials on patients started soon after, but the technique was questioned for its effectiveness and safety and sparked disagreements about research protocols. By 1975, investigation of the use of chymopapain was virtually ended in the United States but the technique continued to be widely used in Canada.

Many American physicians sent their patients to Canada for treatment with chymopapain, preferring that to performing the surgery that would otherwise be the only option. For a time, there was a steady stream of Americans going to Canada for the treatment.

One of these patients, a Palo Alto, Calif., resident, was in a unique position to compare chemonucleolysis with back surgery. Three years before trying chymopapain treatment, he had back surgery for a herniated disk. When the problem recurred, his physician sent him to Vancouver, B.C. for treatment with chymopapain.

"This is definitely the procedure to choose over surgery," he reports. "There is less pain . . . big discomfort for only a day and then just plain discomfort. After surgery, I was in pain for five days and had to stay home five weeks."

The man had the intradiscal therapy on a Friday in Vancouver and flew home to Palo Alto Sunday. He was back at work in a short time and was free of all leg and hip pain.

Physicians feel patients like him are prime candidates for chymopapain, emphasizing it works very well for a specific type of patient. It is considered more useful in relieving leg pain than back pain.

In the United States, two new studies of chymopapain were undertaken in 1980, involving a total of 528 patients. Finally, in early 1983, the U.S. Food and Drug Administration approved the use of chymopapain in the United States. There immediately was a rush of orthopedic surgeons and neurosurgeons to training sessions organized by their specialty medical groups to learn how to perform the new procedure. The interest was so great every session was a sell-out.

The ideal patient for chemonucleolysis is someone with a clear-cut lumbar disk protrusion who suffers constant severe lower-back and leg pain. Conservative treatment, such as bed rest and physical therapy, has produced no improvement for the patient after more than a month's trial.

The same person also is an ideal candidate for surgery. Many physicians are hesitant to get on the chymopapain bandwagon. They feel they have had good results with laminectomies and prefer to continue with the surgery.

In the chemonucleolysis procedure, the patient is taped to a special operating table, lying on his left side with the hips flexed at about a 90-degree angle.

The injection has to be made at a precise location so it is extremely important that the patient is lined up correctly. The position of his spine is checked with a fluoroscopic image intensifier. The doctor can check his movements on the fluoroscopic screen as the procedure continues.

Aside from the delicacy and care that must be used in any technique touching so closely to the spinal cord, the procedure is actually fairly simple. A long needle is inserted into the patient's spine and into the disk. An instructor at one of the training sessions said the sensation he felt as the needle entered the disk was like puncturing a pear.

After the needle is in place, the doctor injects radio-opaque material into the disk to determine its condition. Then the chymopapain powder is reconstituted with sterile water. With the needle in the correct position, the chymopapain is then injected into the disk. More than one disk may be treated at a time.

The procedure may take 45 to 60 minutes, and the needle insertion from 10 to 15 minutes.

The chymopapain, used in the recommended dosages, does not seem to cause any adverse reactions. In about 75 percent of the patients in a double-blind randomized national trial carried out by Smith Laboratories in 1981, the signs and symptoms of a herniated disk were gone within six weeks. Leg pain may continue for a few days after the procedure and back stiffness and soreness may last for several months.

The *Journal of the American Medical Association* reports that a bottle of chymopapain, enough to treat several disks, costs about $525. Physician fees range from $1,200 to $3,000, about the same fees charged for laminectomies.

Nothing is ever perfect and neither is chymopapain. A major risk is that patients may be allergic to the substance; an allergic reaction to chymopapain can cause death.

Because of that risk, chymopapain is used in a hospital setting with an anesthesiologist present. Medication to stop an allergic reaction is already in the syringes, ready to be used in seconds if anything goes wrong. Because of the danger of a patient becoming sensitized to the substance, chymopapain is used only once on a patient.

Hewitt, who formerly sent a number of his patients to Canada, now is using chymopapain in his own practice, and is very happy with the results.

But he feels it's too early to see how chymopapain will change things. The important question, he emphasizes, is whether the procedure will work out well during the long-range period.

Like many other physicians, he worries that chymopapain will be abused and overused, just as laminectomies were after the first ones were performed.

HOT OR COLD: WHICH IS BEST?

What could be more soothing to an aching back than a warm heating pad or hot water bottle?

Surprisingly, a plastic bag of ice cubes may work even better.

Heat has traditionally been recommended to back patients as a way to ease the pain. In some patients, it may still work better.

But cold, perhaps ice cubes in a plastic bag or an ice bag, is being prescribed more often now. Ice is believed to be better than heat in relieving both the pain and inflammation of acute injuries and back pain. Ice is particularly helpful in relieving muscle spasms that may cause such devastating pain in the back.

There are two warnings on the hot/cold front.

First, don't go to bed and sleep on a heating pad all night. You'll wake up worse than when you started. The muscles become so warm and the capillaries so dilated that the spinal column fills up with blood and your back becomes supersensitive.

Secondly, don't get so carried away by the idea cold is good that you turn down the thermostat on your heater, thinking if an ice bag is good a cold house is better. Don't be over-zealous saving on energy costs if you're prone to back problems. A comfortable room temperature is best for your back.

A PAIN IN THE HIP

Many men have the impression that carrying a thick wallet in their hip pocket may cause back problems.

Sitting on your money may indeed cause problems, but not in your back.

It's true that sometimes a thick wallet in the hip pocket has been associated with back and leg pain. But the pain originates in the hip. The wallet may make it slightly worse by causing more pressure on nerves, but it won't touch off a back problem.

Sometimes a wallet or the hammer a carpenter carries on his hip may cause a bursitis from pressure on the nerves. Again, that's in the hip, not the back.

MEDICATION: GOOD OR BAD?

Ordinarily, a patient who goes to his physician complaining of a backache will be given medication to control the pain. The medication may be aspirin or another analgesic or perhaps a muscle relaxant.

For patients with intense pain, stronger medication like morphine may be given.

Doctors, as is true in so many other areas of back treatments, don't agree on the use of pain medication.

One school believes it's important to give the patient pain relief. A doctor explains, "I'm usually generous with pain medication initially. If I can get the patient good and comfortable, it breaks the cycle of pain and apprehension. Then you're a long way ahead. That's why I don't mind subduing a patient, even to the point of making him dopey or sleepy. He won't become addicted in just a few days."

Other physicians prefer not to prescribe much pain medication, claiming it covers the real condition of the patient. They fear a patient with his pain numbed by medication will overdo and further injure his back. However, there is more willingness by these doctors to use a moderate amount of medication as long as the patient is confined to bed.

Drug addicts sometimes hide behind alleged back problems as a way to get narcotics. Their deception is made easier because of the real difficulty of diagnosing back problems.

Patients may come in complaining of severe back pain and asking for medication. The physician can't tell if the complaint is real or not, but if he's suspicious, he will watch carefully.

If the patient calls a few days later, reporting his house was ransacked and the pills disappeared, or that the medication wasn't strong enough and he needs something more powerful, then the physician should immediately refuse to prescribe anything else.

While the physician can't make any accusations without more evidence, he can tell the suspected drug addict, "We don't use narcotics for chronic pain."

SIX:

THE UPPER BACK: A DIFFERENT SITUATION

Most of the time when a reference is made to back problems, it's to lower-back problems because that's the big trouble spot in the spine. The thoracic region at the back of the shoulders is mostly free of problems because there is little movement of vertebrae. The cervical spine in the upper back and neck is flexible, with an even greater range of motion than the lumbar spine.

But the vertebrae and disks in the cervical region have one big advantage over those lower down on the spine. They bear less weight — only the head rather than the head and trunk of the body.

The upper back has its disk problems, but most of its troubles relate to tension more than to slipped disks or weak muscles. However, the neck and cervical region are the risk areas in contact sports. There are a few cases each year of football players becoming paralyzed because of neck injuries.

The risk of injury appears to be greatest in football where the head often is used as a weapon. A player butts another player with his head or hits a player head-on. The head, protected by a helmet, may not suffer much, but the force of the blow is transferred to the neck. There it may cause a shifting of the vertebrae, a pinched nerve or traction on a nerve.

This kind of injury shows up as pain in the arm or muscle weakness. If the pressure is too great, it can cause a fracture and dislocation of the vertebrae. If the nerves are injured to a greater degree, paralysis may result.

Pinched nerves can be treated with rest, muscle strengthening exercises and by wearing a protective collar.

Because the disks age along with the rest of the body, disk problems in the cervical spine are more common in older athletes.

James Cyriax, the British authority on disk problems, believes there are seven progressive stages for disk problems in the cervical region of the spine. Only a few individuals, however, suffer the final stage in which a disk bulges, compressing the dura mater of the spine and perhaps even affecting the spinal cord.

The most common problem of the cervical region is acute torticollis. Also called "wry neck," this ailment most likely affects a person between the ages of 15 and 30. The patient goes to bed normally but next morning finds he can't lift his head off the pillow because of pain radiating from one ear down to the upper shoulder blade area.

Cyriax explains the pain is caused by lying too still for too long a time on a pillow that is too thick or too thin. He suspects it often happens when the victim is away for the weekend, staying with friends or in a hotel, and is given a pillow that's the wrong height for him. He may even have slept soundly without moving his position.

As a result of keeping the neck sideways in one direction all night, the loose fragment of disk shifts its position and jams the joint. When the victim awakes with a crick in his neck, the usual tendency is to complain about sleeping in a draft. The pain may last for a couple days, but goes away on its own accord.

A whiplash injury is another example of a cervical spine problem.

This injury may occur when a car is hit from behind and the driver or passenger is unable to brace himself against it. The head is first thrown backward, then forward, with the unprotected joints bearing the brunt of the force. It usually affects the fifth neck vertebra, where muscles and ligaments can be torn and strained.

The injury is similar to a badly-sprained ankle. The neck should be supported with a protective collar for several weeks. Heat, massage and anti-inflammatory drugs help to relieve symptoms. However, symptoms appear to be aggravated by emotional factors: A tense, anxious person normally takes longer to recover than a relaxed person.

Another cervical problem may occur when there is a block of a cervical joint, causing pain in the shoulder.

Another problem is pressure on a nerve root as it emerges from the spine. The patient may feel severe pain in his arm and a sensation of pins and needles in his fingers for some weeks. The symptoms usually stop spontaneously in three to four months.

Cyriax feels there is a misunderstanding of the normal recovery process in these cases. The patient, unless able to understand the normal course of the problem, gets extremely anxious when nothing the doctor does seems to help. In desperation, the patient may decide to seek another treatment, such as manipulation. It may appear to be successful, when actually it was only that the time of treatment accidentally coincided with the time of normal recovery.

In Cyriax's view, the best way is to explain to the patient the chronological course of the problem and try to keep him comfortable until recovery.

Although cervical disk problems do exist, as much as 70 percent of upper-back pain results from emotional and muscular tension. The neck area feels tension first. Then it's a domino effect: tension moves to the trapezius muscle, which runs in a rough triangle from the back of the skull to the top of the shoulders to the center of the back.

When life becomes too harried, you argue with your employer or you have a marital spat, muscles tense up. Tense muscles are shorter, compressing the nerves and disks in the cervical region.

The person caught in that bind needs to find some way to relax, either by taking a deep breath and consciously slowing down or by trying any one of the common relaxation techniques. If the tension is so constant that cervical pain becomes a problem, biofeedback can be used to help the sufferer train himself to relax.

Psychiatrists get few complaints of lower-back pain from patients. After all, people don't seek counseling when they think their only problem is a back pain.

More often a psychiatrist will hear comments about neck and upper-back pain, even if only in casual references interspersed during conversations about the person's emotional problem.

While some people will respond to tension and stress with a tension headache, others will experience it as a neck pain.

Sometimes the wish, "Get off my back," is translated into an upper-back pain.

SEVEN:

WHAT ELSE CAN GO WRONG?

Back problems involving muscles, tension or disks are the most common, but by no means are the whole picture.

Remember, more than 100 diagnoses can be made for back pain and that represents a host of other problems. Sometimes the back pain is a symptom of illness in another part of the body, perhaps in the kidneys. A tumor also may be developing on the spine.

Following is an alphabetical listing of some other disorders that may affect the back.

ANKYLOSING SPONDYLITIS

Ankylosing spondylitis or spinal arthritis is the disease that in its extreme form causes the stiff poker back.

Most forms of arthritis inflame only the inside of the joints. But ankylosing spondylitis also causes inflammation of the ligaments and of the outsides of the joints. In addition, the inflammation can cause a bony overgrowth on the spine, fusing it solid.

The first joints usually affected are the sacroiliac joints which link the base of the spine to the pelvis. Bony growths fuse the normally separate bones together. The problem may move up the spine until it affects many or possibly all of the joints between the vertebrae.

The disease generally starts fairly early in life, with symptoms appearing by the late teens or early 20s. Back pain may awake the victim during the night, with the pain relieved by light exercise.

Other possible symptoms are vague chest pains and general fatigue. For reasons not clearly understood, the disease also may cause the eyes to become red and painful. Severe cases may cause stiffness in the spinal column forcing the head to permanently bend over onto the chest.

However, for most people, the disease does not become that severe. A good exercise routine and use of anti-inflammatory drugs can keep it under control. Often the doctor will prescribe drugs to be used prophylactically, such as before skiing, when the person knows his back will be subjected to more stress.

BACK SPRAIN

Back sprain is a common diagnosis for lower-back problems, sort of a catch-all word similar to "lumbago" which is still popularly used in England.

Most often, however, when people refer to problems caused by a sprained back, the pain and discomfort actually is produced by a disk problem or a degenerative condition.

Sometimes the term "back sprain" is accurate if it refers to an acute stretching of muscles and tendons causing them to tear, just as in a sprained ankle.

But experts consider it a myth that back sprain accounts for a large number of back problems. As with a sprained ankle, a sprained back will heal itself, although the pain may linger for a while.

BROKEN OR
FRACTURED BACK

Backbones can be broken or fractured just like leg or wrist bones. An accident of some sort or sudden pressure can fracture a vertebrae. At the same time, the blow that crushes the vertebrae may also pressure the intervertebral disk.

Many times there will be small stress fractures that the person doesn't even realize have occurred. These fractures often happen in an elderly person or perhaps in a gymnast or athlete who challenges his body to the utmost.

With a serious fracture, extreme care should be taken because there is always the danger that the spinal cord may be affected. A tragedy could result if the person is moved by a well-intentioned rescuer unaware of the risks. Don't move or lift the patient until medical help arrives. Never try to lift him into your car to rush him to the hospital.

Suspect a broken neck or back if the patient has had a bad fall, a whiplash-type neck injury or has been in any accident where the back or neck is bent or struck. If the victim is conscious but unable to move his hands or fingers, he may have a neck fracture. If he cannot move his feet and toes, suspect a back fracture.

With rest, fractured vertebrae in the back will heal gradually and back pain usually goes away.

Severe fractures are fairly uncommon, but small stress fractures occur quite frequently. They are difficult to recognize on an X-ray and the diagnosis is often missed. These small fractures may occur in the vertebral arches at the back of the spinal column because this part of the spine normally transmits a large proportion of the total force. Often back pain may be blamed on another reason when actually caused by a small fracture.

CERVICAL
SPONDYLOSIS

Cervical spondylosis affects the seven vertebrae in the cervical or upper back and neck region of the spinal column and the disks that act as cushions between them.

Bony outgrowths develop on the vertebrae and there may be a misalignment or a hardening of the disks. The neck becomes stiff and an abnormal amount of pressure is exerted on the nerve pathways in the upper part of the spine, especially those running between the spinal cord and the arms and hands.

The cause of cervical spondylosis is unknown but it is more prevalent among the middle-aged and elderly perhaps because some bones tend to become knobby and irregular as people age. Men and women are equally susceptible to the disease.

A stiff neck is the main symptom. There also may be pain and tingling or numbness in the shoulders or arms.

Pressure within the neck may in time affect other portions of the spinal cord, perhaps causing a gradual weakening of the legs or problems with bladder control. Blood vessels that run through cervical vertebrae to the brain may become constricted, causing symptoms such as headache, dizziness, unsteadiness or double vision, especially if the patient tries to bend his neck.

Cervical spondylosis is a common disorder. If the symptoms are minor, people experience discomfort but do not need to see a doctor. In most cases the symptoms do not get worse; but in very severe cases, the lower half of the body may become paralyzed.

If the minor symptoms persist and seem to be getting worse, a physician should be consulted. He may order either an X-ray or a myelogram to determine the extent of the pressure on the spinal cord.

The bothersome symptoms are best treated by having the patient wear a supportive collar. Collars prevent extreme movements of the neck, holding it in a position to minimize pressure on the cervical nerves and blood vessels. The collar is usually worn for several months, and often there are no further problems. Analgesics or pain killers also may be used. The physician may prescribe a tranquilizer to relax the patient and keep the neck muscles from tightening.

If the symptoms get worse it may be necessary to use traction to relieve the problem or to have an operation. A surgeon can enlarge the constricted bony canal or fuse together some of the cervical vertebrae or both. These procedures give relief from the symptoms but limit the ability to turn or bend the neck.

FEET AND LEG PROBLEMS

Conditions in the feet and legs also can be a factor in back problems.

A fallen arch in the foot may cause the leg to turn inward, resulting in possible tension on the sciatic nerve. If there is more of a collapse in one foot than the other the effect is the same as one leg being shorter than the other.

The same situation occurs when one leg actually is shorter, creating an imbalance in the way muscles are used and causing back pain.

Usually these conditions are not difficult to correct. An orthotic device in the shoe will solve arch problems and a lift in one shoe can equalize the leg lengths.

Sometimes people complain of pain in their back after being fitted with an orthotic device by a podiatrist. This condition is caused as the back muscles are retrained to a new way of moving. Podiatrists suggest patients break into wearing an orthotic device gradually, giving their muscles a chance to adjust.

MUSCLE SPASMS

An acute case of back pain sometimes is caused by a muscle spasm, an involuntary and sustained contraction of a muscle in the back.

Sometimes, in a person who is constantly too tense, the back muscles can be in chronic spasm. Other times, an acute spasm serves as a protective mechanism, contracting the muscle into sort of a protective splint. Or, if a muscle is injured or over-strained, neighboring muscles may go into spasm to protect it.

Spasms can be extremely painful. Although muscles aren't tender in their normal state, they become sensitive and painful when swollen by the tension of spasm.

The pain of muscle spasm results from a lack of nutrition. When the muscle contracts, the capillaries that supply blood are cut off and oxygen and blood can't reach the muscle cells. Also, waste products can't be removed. These waste products, which include lactic acid, can produce pain when they accumulate in a muscle.

A muscle in spasm feels hard and knotty, its motion restricted. A spasm in a neck muscle, for instance, may make it impossible to bend the neck enough to place the chin on the shoulder.

It's possible to determine if muscles in your back are in spasm by having a friend or family member knead your back gently with his fingertips or the heel of his hand. If there is tenderness when the hand presses gently, that particular muscle is in spasm.

Relaxation techniques, a gentle massage or perhaps soothing heat are helpful in reducing muscle spasms.

OSTEOARTHRITIS

Osteoarthritis is a degenerative disorder of the joints, often called wear and tear arthritis or degenerative arthritis.

It's a condition that develops normally as a result of wear and tear on the joints, and shows up most frequently in older people.

Osteoarthritis causes the smooth lining of the joint, called the articular cartilage, to crack or flake from overuse, injury or some other reason. As the cartilage deteriorates, the underlying bone may become thickened or distorted. These degenerative changes can affect the small facet joints that lie behind and on either side of the vertebral canal.

The earliest changes may show up in the 30-year-old group, and by 60, almost everybody shows some wear and tear on their spine.

Osteoarthritis may cause episodes of mild discomfort and the pain may become severe enough to interfere with daily life. As the joints continue to degenerate and become stiffer and immobile, it may become less painful.

Osteoarthritis occurs so frequently it might be labeled a common cause for backaches. However, this theory has not been proven. In surveys comparing the evidence of wear and tear on the spine with the incidence of backache, there was only a small difference in the frequency of backache between patients with good X-rays and those with the worst X-rays.

Normally, self-help measures are sufficient for persons with osteoarthritis. An occasional dose of aspirin and keeping warm helps to ease most joint pains. If the problems become more severe, the physician may recommend anti-inflammatory drugs or steroids.

OSTEOPOROSIS

Osteoporosis, a disorder principally associated with aging, causes thinning of the bones. The bones lose mass and become brittle, making victims highly vulnerable to fractures.

In healthy bone, chemistry is balanced between the breakdown of old bone tissue and the manufacture of new bone. In osteoporosis, breakdown occurs faster than replacement and the bones become soft and weak.

The ailment is getting increased attention now as a larger segment of the population reaches the older age range.

More than 10 million post-menopausal women in the United States suffer from osteoporosis. Medical complications cost more than $4 billion annually.

Osteoporosis produces back pain from fractures of the vertebrae. In advanced cases, it may lead to an exaggerated "hunchback." The disease also may cause loss of height and contributes to an estimated 200,000 hip fractures a year.

Osteoporosis usually doesn't produce symptoms unless it occurs in the spinal column. Then a person may notice he is becoming shorter and more round-shouldered due to the gradual compression of weakened vertebrae. In rare cases, one or several vertebrae may collapse, causing a sudden, extremely severe attack of back pain.

There are no specific treatments for osteoporosis, although some medical experts feel a woman is better protected if she takes estrogen hormones for a period during and after menopause.

It is generally thought also that exercise is helpful in preventing the development of osteoporosis. A good physical fitness program throughout life may help avoid osteoporosis. Nutrition also may be a factor.

The loss of bone mass also can occur in people confined to bed for long periods of time and in astronauts who spend time in the weightlessness of outer space.

Recently, the disorder has been found in other groups of people. They include young women who exercise so vigorously they cease menstruating, alcoholic men, premenopausal women whose ovaries have been removed, and asthma, allergy and arthritis sufferers who take cortoid steroids.

Modified scanner. Researchers at the University of California, San Francisco, currently are studying the problem. They are using a pioneering technique that involves modifying a CAT scanner, which produces a cross-section image of the body, to get quantitative density information from a scan of a patient.

Rather than just taking the picture, the modified scanner is able to analyze the amount of bone mineral present and whether there is some degree of osteoporosis.

The modified CAT scanner provides a sensitive tool for detecting which women are losing bone mass fast and which risk developing fractures, and for testing the effectiveness of various medications.

Studies. The researchers hope to detect and monitor osteoporosis in patients so that it doesn't continue on to complications.

In 1982, the UCSF researchers published the results of a study of osteoporosis in women who had had their ovaries removed. The three-year study of 37 women ranging in age from 24 to 49 found that on average they lost spinal bone mass at an "alarmingly" rapid rate, nine percent a year after the operation. Administering low-dosage estrogen produced very encouraging results, not only stopping bone loss but also causing a number of women to regain substantial amounts of bone mass.

The researchers presently are involved in a three-year study of 120 women just beginning menopause to establish the natural rate of loss in spinal mass when menstruation ceases and to assess which of several medications is most effective in slowing or halting the rate of loss.

They also are making a study of women track teams at Stanford University and University of California, Berkeley, and of running clubs to substantiate findings of dramatic bone loss in athletic women who have stopped menstruating.

SCHEURMANN'S DISEASE

Scheurmann's disease, sometimes called "adolescent's round back," is a disorder in which growth changes in the thoracic vertebrae to give them a wedge-shaped formation increasing the thoracic curve.

The disorder usually occurs in teen-agers and is a common cause of back pain in this age group. The active state of the disease may last from two to five years.

Scheurmann's disease is self-limiting and not serious, although there is a possibility it will cause an undesirable deformity.

Treatment usually calls only for limitation of activity and back muscle exercises. In more severe cases, it may be necessary to prescribe bed rest, followed by the wearing of a spinal brace. In rare cases, a surgical fusion may be necessary.

SCIATICA

Sciatica is the term for pain in the lower body and legs caused when a problem in the back presses on the sciatic nerve, the largest of all nerves. It branches from the spine throughout the lower body and legs.

Sciatica is most often caused by a rupture in a disk of the spine, which causes pressure on the nerve root. Depending on the severity of the cause, the pain may be felt in the lower back or part-way down the leg or it may go so far as to cause numbness and tingling in the toes.

Usually, in sciatica, the pain runs down the back of the thigh, the back or the outside of the lower leg and the outer edge or the top of the foot. Sometimes it is difficult for people to describe where the pain is located, but somewhat easier to describe the location of the tingling sensations.

The pain is made worse by straining, coughing or sneezing; these actions raise the pressure within the vertebral canal and add slightly to the stress on the nerves.

One of the tests physicians use to detect sciatica is straight-leg raising. The patient lies on his back and the doctor raises the ankle as far as possible with the knee held out straight. This test presents no problem for the normal person, but for someone with sciatica, the movement is severely limited. Straight-leg raising stretches the sciatic nerve and pulls on the nerve root, making the pain even more severe.

Treatment of underlying disk problems will produce improvement in sciatica. The improvement can be measured by repeating the straight leg raising test to check if pain-free motion has been restored.

SCOLIOSIS

The spine normally has a forward/backward S-shaped curve for flexibility and shock-absorbing qualities.

Sometimes the spine develops a lateral curvature, a condition called scoliosis. There are many types of scoliosis, but the most common is called idiopathic scoliosis (meaning there is no known cause).

This type of scoliosis usually appears between the ages of eight and 13, and strikes young girls most often. It may be caused by either faulty bone structure or inadequate supporting muscles. The curve is usually to the right in the chest region and to the left in the lower-back area.

A national survey estimated scoliosis occurs in about 2.4 million adolescent and pre-adolescent Americans. Most cases are mild and can't be detected except in examinations by someone trained in the field or by X-rays. About 15 percent of all cases are severe enough to cause disfiguration; very severe cases can lead to heart and lung damage.

Diagnosis. Scoliosis may be difficult for parents to detect in their children. Often an opposing curvature will form as the body tries to compensate and the child will continue to appear to stand straight. Many times the only indication is a slight deviation in posture. One hip may appear slightly higher or fuller than the other or one shoulder may appear slightly higher. With opposing curvatures of equal size, the only way scoliosis can be detected is when the child bends over a lump becomes visible on part of the back.

Many schools have started screening programs to search out cases of scoliosis. School nurses or physical education teachers are trained to do the screening.

Treatment. Treatment for scoliosis is a combination of exercise, bracing and surgical fusion, depending on the type and severity of the problem.

Two new methods of treatment also are being tried. One uses direct electrical stimulation of the spine muscles during sleep. The other is an augmented feedback plastic brace that reminds the child to shift the trunk at regular intervals during the day. If the cause of idiopathic scoliosis is abnormal neuromusclar control, this new brace could be particularly effective.

The more conventional treatment is to fit the child with a hip-to-neck brace that holds the spine straight. The brace is worn 23 hours a day or less, depending on the severity of the curvature. The brace is worn usually from one to two years or longer. A brace can be used as a corrective treatment only while the patient is still growing. After that, it's ineffective.

Wearing a brace may sound like a simple treatment for a potentially crippling ailment, but it's not that easy.

The brace is prescribed just at a time when the young patients are growing and developing and are extremely sensitive to what their friends will think. Some young scoliosis patients refuse to wear their braces or are in constant conflict with their parents over the devices.

Efforts are being made in some areas to counteract this situation by establishing support groups for young scoliosis patients. These groups help the patients realize they are not alone and encourage the youngsters adopt a "Let's live life and wear a brace, too" attitude.

Not all curvatures of the spine are serious enough to warrant wearing a brace. One problem facing doctors is to determine which cases need treatment and which can go unchecked.

SPINA BIFIDA

Spina bifida is a congenital irregularity of the spine: The bony part of the spine protecting the spinal cord fails to develop properly. The nerves of the spinal cord are left exposed and unprotected in that area, usually in the lower spine.

The spinal nerves in that area control the muscles of the legs, bladder and bowels. Consequently, a child born with the disorder may have some paralysis in his legs and may be unable to control the bladder and bowels.

There is a wide range in the severity of the defect in the base of the spine and the damage to the spinal cord. In some cases, the only evidence may be a small dimple in the skin over the baby's spine. Other babies with the disorder may have a large purplish-red membrane on their backs that covers a gap in the spine.

However, a common form of spina bifida, called spina bifida occulta, may affect as many as 25 percent of the population.

Usually it causes no problems, although it may result in lower-back pain where muscles attach somewhat off center because of the opening, putting an added strain on them.

For severe cases in infants, surgery may be performed to repair the membrane on the child's back. However, little can be done to correct any nerve damage.

SPINAL CORD INJURIES

Injuries to the spine also may damage the spinal cord as it passes through the spinal column in a canal protected by vertebrae and disks.

The nerve pathways that make up the spinal cord transmit impulses between the brain and all parts of the body. If the spinal cord is damaged by an accident, part or parts of the body below the injury may be affected.

Spinal cord injuries are very common today because of auto and motorcycle accidents, sports injuries and gunshot wounds.

An injury to the spinal cord in the neck can be fatal if it damages the nerves that control breathing. This kind of injury can totally paralyze both arms and legs and cause numbness from the neck down.

Injuries to other parts of the spinal cord are not fatal, but can cause permanent paralysis.

Symptoms. Symptoms of spinal cord injury almost always appear immediately after the injury. They depend on the location of the damage to the spinal cord. There may be numbness or weakness or paralysis of all muscles below the level of the injury, although sometimes only muscles on one side of the body are affected. Pain is not always a symptom although sometimes injury to nearby muscles will cause pain.

Serious injury to the spinal cord always requires immediate hospitalization. As with a possible back fracture, don't try to move the patient — wait for trained medical personnel. As soon as possible the patient's spine will be X-rayed to determine the extent of

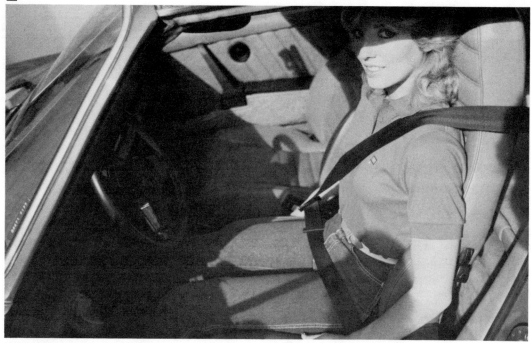

Wearing a seat belt while driving can help you avoid dangerous spinal cord injuries.

damage, and a myelogram may be performed to see if it may be possible to relieve pressure on the spinal cord by surgery.

Treatment. This kind of problem is truly a case where the best treatment is prevention.

Never dive into water head first unless you're sure how deep it is. If you must jump in, do it feet first. You still might break your back but at least you won't break your neck.

Other tips: wear seat belts while driving, don't drink or use drugs and drive, and use normal care in climbing stairs and walking on slippery surfaces.

The spinal cord patient who is a paraplegic or quadraplegic faces months in a hospital and in rehabilitation units to help him adapt to life in his changed situation.

SPINAL STENOSIS

Spinal stenosis is a narrowing of the vertebral canal which protects the spinal cord and nerve roots.

The shape and size of these canals can vary considerably. If someone is born with a small canal, there is more of a chance that disk protrusions will press against the nerves, causing back pain.

Spinal stenosis occurs in about 15 percent of the population. Usually the spine is narrow at birth, but occasionally, bony thickening develops around the disk borders and the facet joints, or for some other reason the canal is narrowed.

People with this condition are considered more of a risk to develop sciatica (see page 57).

Symptoms. A characteristic set of symptoms accompanies spinal stenosis. The patient may develop lower-back pain with numbness, tingling and cramps in the lower leg. These symptoms may develop after walking only a few hundred yards and may be sufficiently severe to force the patient to stop and rest. After five or 10 minutes, the pain lessens because the flood of blood within the vertebral canal during exercise may cause even more pressure against the already tightly-packed nerve roots.

Because the physical dimensions of the vertebral canal are slightly larger when the spine is bent forward than when bent backward, there may be less discomfort when the person bends forward. Walking may present symptoms, but a person with spinal stenosis may be able to bicycle without problems because in cycling, he leans forward.

Treatment. The same therapies used for other lower back problems caused by slipped disks may be applied in cases of spinal stenosis. Sometimes it may be possible surgically to eliminate the narrowing.

SPONDYLOSIS

Just as osteoarthritis causes degenerative changes in the spine, another disorder called spondylosis reflects wear and tear on the disks.

The disks start out as springy cushions with a jelly-like center. With age, they become tough and fibrous, losing some of their vertical height. No longer are they the same resilient cushions.

At the same time, the bony surfaces above and below the disks begin to show wear and tear. The surfaces of the bone thicken and a rim of bone develops around the edge of the disk.

Along with those changes, bony growths may develop on the vertebrae or along the edge of the degenerating disks. These growths may press painfully on various nerves where they join the spinal cord.

Spondylosis often accompanies osteoarthritis. Sometimes, it is difficult to distinguish which disorder is causing the symptoms. Mild cases of spondylosis are usually symptom-free. A person can have the disease without knowing it.

More severe cases can cause intermittent pain in the part of the back that is most seriously affected, usually the lower back. The back may become increasingly tender and difficult to bend or twist. Spondylosis in the lower back may cause shooting pains in the buttocks and legs if there is pressure on the sciatic nerve.

SPONDYLOLISTHESIS

Spondylolisthesis is a disorder of the spine in which a forward displacement of a lower-back vertebra is caused by a bony defect between the vertebra and the arch enclosing the spinal cord. As a result, there is a degeneration of the disk.

The disorder can exist without symptoms and may be discovered accidently during a routine physical examination. The defect may be congenital or it may develop early in life. Speculation is that the disorder is set off by tiny stress fractures that occur from the frequent bumping and bouncing an infant goes through as he learns to walk.

When symptoms occur, they are usually lower-back ache and possibly leg pain. Treatment is the same as for a disk lesion.

Many teen-agers and young adults lead normal lives, despite having spondylolisthesis.

TRIGGER POINTS

A trigger point is usually an area so small it can be covered by a fingertip. Any area larger is probably either a muscle spasm or a muscle spasm surrounding a trigger point.

Trigger points are small areas of tenderness in the back. Biopsies show some evidence of chronic inflammatory cells, but little is really understood about the exact composition of a trigger point.

The phenomenon of trigger points was discovered shortly before World War II. They were given that name because pressing on these little areas can ''trigger'' or set off pain in another area.

Some physicians feel that, whatever the mechanism of the trigger point, treatment of it can result in dramatic relief from pain. Treatment usually consists of injections of anesthetics and cortisone.

It's interesting to note that in many instances the location of trigger points coincides with acupuncture sites.

EIGHT:

YOUR BACK HURTS: WHAT NOW?

Your back hurts. Maybe it's a dull ache that's been nagging at you for a couple weeks. Perhaps you reached for something on the rear seat of your car, suddenly felt a sharp stab of pain and could barely straighten up.

Whatever happened, you realize there's a problem and it's time to do something about it.

The sensible reaction is to phone your family doctor. There are so many things that could possibly cause a back problem, it makes sense to start with a family-practice specialist or a primary-care physician who can recommend whatever specialist might be needed. However, many patients prefer going directly to a specialist, perhaps an orthopedic surgeon.

THE BACK EXAM

You make an appointment and go to the doctor's office. What happens then?

Normally, the procedure would be pretty much like that followed by Dr. Myron Gananian, a family-practice physician at the Palo Alto Medical Foundation.

There might be a difference, though. Gananian has had problems with his own back which he feels gives him a special empathy with back patients. While many physicians are frustrated by the vagueness of back problems and the difficulty of achieving clear-cut cures, Gananian is intrigued by them, and enjoys treating back patients.

Gananian believes his own disk trouble started because he may have overdone some stretching exercises. He's since been able to return to running and weight lifting with no problems. In fact, the only time his back has bothered him was when he set off on a drive to Los Angeles. Within an hour, he was feeling back pain.

He feels generally he can do just about any sports activity now, but believes it's better for his back if he plans a variety of activities rather than concentrating on just one sport.

Gananian has found that the point at which patients come in to see him depends on their personality and what else is going on in their lives. Some patients will come in within two days of the onset of pain; others will put up with pain for a month or more before calling for an appointment.

They may complain of a dull or a sharp pain, but usually what brings them in is that they can't function. If the back problem interferes with their normal activity, such as driving a car or bending over a microscope, then that brings them to the doctor's office.

The routine of the examination may vary, depending on the patient's personality and problem, but it more or less follows this sequence:

HISTORY

First, a history is taken to find out if the problem started with an injury or if similar pain had occurred previously.

Questions may include: When did the pain start and was the onset sudden or gradual? How is the general health of the patient? What is his conditioning or exercise level? What kind of work does he do? Has there been a recent weight gain? Is the person taking any medicine that might conflict with what the doctor might prescribe? Is the patient taking pills for high blood pressure? (They could cause a mineral imbalance that might have some bearing on what's going on in the back.)

OBSERVATION

Gananian also carefully watches the way a patient moves. The patient should be unclothed so the doctor can see the back and lower extremities and note the posture. He will have the patient walk to check gait. He watches carefully to see how the patient gets up on the examination table.

"If the patient jumps up on it, as if he were jumping on a horse or climbing a fence, you know he is not in discomfort," Gananian says. "If he kind of creeps up and approaches the table like it was the gas chamber, you know he either is faking or is in a lot of pain."

If a patient comes in with pain going down his leg, which indicates there is nerve involvement, an X-ray may be ordered.

Gananian also will make further checks to see if there appears to be nerve involvement. A patient who has pain down his leg and who feels more pain in his back and leg with a deep breath may have a disk pressing on a sciatic nerve. The patient's reflexes will be checked by tapping the knee. Also, a vibrating tuning fork may be placed on the ankle or big toe. The patient's ability to feel or not feel the vibrations is a sensitive indicator of the presence or absence of disk problems.

Another test is to have the person close his eyes and then move the big toe on one foot. People with disk problems lose their ability to tell what position the toe is in.

DIAGNOSIS

If the patient shows any of these signs, indicating a significant disk involvement, Gananian tends to refer them immediately to a specialist, either to an orthopedic surgeon or neurosurgeon, or, if the problem seems to be primarily a nerve one, to a neurologist.

His reasoning is that two weeks in bed may not help these patients. The specialist may make the same initial recommendation of bed rest, but Gananian feels it's best if the specialist gets in the act early. That way the specialist has a chance to evaluate the patient in the initial stages of the problem. If bed rest doesn't help, the specialist is already familiar with the case and more prepared to decide on a next step of treatment.

In trying to diagnose back problems, the primary-care physician also has to rule out non-spine reasons for the pain. Usually, an X-ray will tell if there is possible cancer of the bone or of the breast.

For patients in their 30s or 40s, the chances of finding a surprise on the X-ray is not too likely, Gananian says. A 35-year-old woman with a backache is unlikely to have breast cancer. But if it's a 60-year-old woman, cancer is something worth considering early.

Gananian's examination also will seek to determine whether the back pain is caused by kidney problems.

TREATMENT

If the conclusion is that the problem is a fairly routine form of back disorder, he will start the patient on a conservative regimen of treatment.

If the patient is having a lot of back pain, Gananian recommends bed rest for a week or so, with the patient being permitted up only to eat and go to the bathroom. He hasn't put a patient in the hospital for traction for a long time, believing bed rest can do the same thing at home without the expensive hospitalization.

"If the patient is good for the first couple or three days, he can increase gradually the duration of time he is up and around,'' Gananian says. ''Some of the patients go to bed for a day or two and are better.''

The specialists also repeat the same type of basic examination when they first see patients. Always, it's important for them to get a sense of how the patient moves and how much discomfort he is in.

The orthopedic surgeons and neurosurgeons at the Palo Alto Medical Foundation are trained to perform surgery on back patients if necessary. But they prefer to start with conservative treatments, using surgery or the newer chemonucleolysis only as a last resort.

Another specialist who might see a back patient is a rheumatologist, an expert on arthritic and rheumatic problems in the back. Such a specialist also would be the first choice if the patient is suspected of having ankylosing spondylitis, an arthritic condition seen most often in young men.

A sports medicine expert also might get into the picture if the back problem seems related to athletic activities. He would analyze back problems caused by muscles, particularly if an athlete had stressed his muscles the wrong way.

Because of the specialist's knowledge of how the body acts in sports, he can understand, for example, how running in the wrong position may cause lower-back pain. Running with the chest over-expanded can cause an excessive swayback position straining the back. Conversely, running with the trunk thrust forward also can cause back problems.

Swimmers may show up in the sports medicine physician's office. Sometimes they spend a lot of time doing one thing, such as putting a float board in front of them and kicking. That causes the same kind of exaggerated swayback. Golfers, however, rarely report back pain.

The sports medicine specialist is able to treat the patient for the problem that brought him in and also advise him on how to prevent a recurrence.

PHYSICAL THERAPY

All of the above mentioned physicians may refer the patient to the physical therapy department. The physicians have evaluated the patient, relying on their knowledge and on X-ray and neurological tests. By the time a patient is referred to the physical therapy department, a diagnosis has been made and treatment started.

Physical therapy is one of the ways to both treat the patient and to help insure he doesn't become a back pain victim again.

After the doctor gives the physical therapist his impressions, the therapist evaluates the patient based on what physical therapy has to offer. The patient will be put through a range of movements — bending forward and backward, then to the side, rotating the spine one way and the other — to get an idea of what the problem is.

A patient with a disk problem feels pain when he bends forward while a facet joint problem will cause discomfort if the patient bends backward.

Tami King, a physical therapist at the Palo Alto Medical Foundation, compares a facet joint problem to a finger jammed backward. Just as the finger will hurt if it is pushed farther backward, it will hurt an already irritated facet joint if the spine is bent backward and more pressure placed on the joint.

Disk and facet joint problems will give totally different signs. Bending forward will make a facet problem feel better and a disk problem feel worse. Bending to the side of the pain will make a facet problem worse.

The physical therapist also will evaluate whether the back problem is caused by muscle strain.

In the past, most physical therapists had only a standard set of exercises, called Williams exercises, to give to all patients. With the flush of new knowledge that has been developed in recent years, there's been a great change.

Better understanding of disk problems and new forms of exercise and therapy developed by a New Zealand physiotherapist, Robin McKenzie, have made a tremendous difference. Now it's possible to prescribe exercises specifically designed to correct a particular back problem.

Someone with disk problems will be given exercises based on McKenzie's theory that bending backward helps realign the disks and spine into a correct position.

A patient with problems in the facet joints, the small joints alongside the vertebrae in the spine, will get exercises calling for forward bending movements.

The therapist also prescribes exercises to take care of other muscle groups that play a role in back problems. Abdominal muscles should be strengthened; hamstring, groin muscles and heel cords stretched.

The physical therapist also does manipulations and mobilizations that patients can't do on their own.

Mobilizations are passive movements of the joint to restore mobility. In manipulations, the therapist will move a joint manually, pushing on different parts of it to cause movements of a particular segment of the spine.

Stretching and massage also are forms of treatment.

An important aspect of physical therapy is teaching a patient how to move, sit and lift so the back problem doesn't recur.

"A patient comes in and you do all these wonderful things, King comments. "But if you don't teach them that first day how to sit and how to get out of bed, the basic body mechanics to get them through to when they come back to you, they can go home and undo all you've done.

"Patient education is the most important thing a physical therapist can do, she continues. "You can relieve all the spasms and get rid of the inflammation and pain . . . but in three weeks, six months or a year, if they continue to do these things, their backs are going to wear down and go out again."

She finds patients may be cocky after the first episode of back pain is over and quickly forget how painful their back was.

"But as soon as a little back pain starts to creep in, you say, 'Oh, no,' and start doing your exercises again, she notes. "After the second time that happens, exercises become a part of your life.

"If you're smart, you catch on. Otherwise, you'll be back here every six months or a year."

OTHER TREATMENTS

Back complaints and back patients are so individual that a wide range of treatments may provide relief to some patients and may particularly appeal to them.

Some treatments are new developments, such as the back schools that teach people how to live happily with their backs.

Others are older activities, such as yoga and the Alexander Technique, which advocates believe can play an important role in helping people alleviate their back problems.

These are a few of the possibilities you might want to examine as alternative ways to cope with back problems:

ACUPUNCTURE

Almost everyone now is familiar with acupuncture, the traditional Chinese medical technique.

Although there is no scientific evidence documenting how it works, the Chinese have been using the procedure successfully for 3000 years and it recently has become popular in the United States. Many M.D.s have studied the technique so they can offer it as a choice to their patients.

The Chinese believe that energy, called "chi," circulates all through the universe under the control of opposite forces called yin and yang.

In the human body, the belief is that energy flows along 12 parallel lines or meridians running the length of the body and its extremities. Most meridian lines are associated with major body organs.

After a diagnosis of an imbalance of energy flow, an acupuncturist will insert thin needles in any of 500 to 1000 points along the meridian. Acupuncture, used most often for pain, theoretically works by adjusting the energy flow along the meridians.

Scientific studies of the use of acupuncture in treating lower-back problems, reported in the *Journal of the American Medical Association,* indicate no significant effectiveness of the therapy. However, many people claim they have felt benefits from acupuncture, and the subjective feeling of relief is terribly important to a suffering back patient.

ALEXANDER TECHNIQUE

The Alexander Technique was developed more than half a century ago by an Australian, Matthias Alexander.

Alexander was a successful Shakespearean actor, but was plagued increasingly by voice trouble. His stage career was ended by his recurrent loss of voice.

In desperation, he decided to study how he used muscles as he spoke, in an effort to determine which movements might be related to the loss of his voice. He found the most troublesome movement consisted of tightening the head backward on the neck and downward into the chest.

Correcting that movement, which Alexander believed led to many of the muscle and postural problems experienced by people, is still the keystone of the technique. Interestingly, it is having a modern day emergence in the teachings of physical therapists who also believe head position is important to correct body posture.

Many actors and performers study the Alexander Technique. For example, it is taught at the noted American Conservatory Theater in San Francisco.

Many Alexander Technique students are people with back problems or muscular problems, such as violinists who may develop trouble because of the position they must maintain while playing.

The technique is relevant to back problems because the wrong movement of the head and neck, so criticized by Alexander, may be a factor in back pain. Tightening the head backward and downward into the chest creates both tension and pressure on the spine.

Essentially, the technique teaches correct ways to move the body in daily activities, always with an emphasis on the correct position of the head. Teachers of the technique also stress the importance of a serene, unhurried approach to life.

BACK SCHOOLS

The concept of back schools was originated in the late 1950s by Dr. Harry Fahrni of Vancouver, B.C., who developed an education program for his patients. He believed back pain was controllable and developed body mechanics techniques to help the back stay in good health.

Ten years later, a Swedish back school was organized at a Volvo motor plant to treat industrial patients. The school proved successful in getting Volvo workers back on the job.

Now, there are hundreds of back schools in the United States. Patient questionnaires reveal 95 percent of the graduates have been able, with instruction on spinal mechanics and exercise routines, to keep pain down to an acceptable level for years.

A back school typically will evaluate a student, determining what his problem is and how he can be helped. By using a school concept, it is possible to teach more students at a time than could be done by a physical therapist giving a patient individual attention.

The school may offer a series of several classes in which the student is instructed in correct ways of sitting, lifting and working, as well as sports activities.

Many industries now are organizing back schools for their employees. In one program, 39,000 employees of Southern Pacific Transportation Co. attended a back school. Safeway Stores also has instituted a back school program. By teaching its employees how to use straight back bending in loading and unloading objects from low shelves, Safeway was able to reduce the incidence of its employees' most frequent back injuries.

CHIROPRACTIC

Chiropractic does not use drugs or surgery and is not intended specifically to treat disease. Instead, the theory of chiropractic is that the structural and functional integrity of the nervous system is maintained by massage, spinal manipulations and adjustment of joints and soft tissues.

Many back patients go to chiropractors when they feel their medical doctor is not helping their problem. Most often, they will be treated with heat, massage and sometimes with manipulations.

Medical doctors are skeptical of much that is done in chiropractic, questioning whether the manipulation techniques are based on accurate knowledge of the spine.

However, some patients do report relief after a manipulation, although that relief may coincide with the natural spontaneous recovery that occurs with many back problems.

One physician comments that chiropractic is basically a form of physical therapy and does relieve some people. However, he objects to the fact chiropractors tend to encourage patients to return all the time. However, he concedes that steady treatment might be the biggest benefit to the patient who perceives that his doctor is not doing enough for him.

"There's not much back patients can do but rest," he notes, "but some patients want to have hands laid on."

MYOTHERAPY

Myotherapy was developed by Bonnie Prudden, a leading authority on physical fitness and exercise therapy who was instrumental in helping create the President's

Council on Physical Fitness and Sports in the 1950s. She presently is director of the Institute for Physical Fitness and Myotherapy in Stockbridge, Mass.

Myotherapy is designed to ease pain by pressure on trigger points, the sensitive painful points in muscles where they may have been "damaged" by stress or spasm.

Among the people who inspired Prudden to develop myotherapy was Dr. Hans Kraus, noted back authority. Kraus came to her aid one morning when she was planning a mountain climb but woke up with a painful, stiff neck. Kraus used strong pressure with his thumb to press on a trigger point in her neck and Prudden was relieved immediately. She also was inspired by Dr. Janet Travell, White House physician under Presidents Johnson and Kennedy, who had developed a procedure for injecting trigger points.

Prudden confidently claims backache is the easiest pain to ease with myotherpay.

The technique calls for applying pressure to trigger points located in a region that corresponds to the "back pockets of their blue jeans." Pressure is applied with a bent elbow, angled back to the person giving the therapy. It is possible to locate the trigger points because the pressure will bring a pain response immediately.

The same technique also is applied to trigger points higher up on the back.

Stretching and limbering exercises are then prescribed to relax the back muscles.

SELF-HELP

The trend in popular medicine today is toward self-help. People want to be in charge of their own bodies and to take responsibility for their own health care.

That feeling is adaptable to the back patient. Many back problems can be prevented or cured by what the patient can do on his own. In fact, even if a patient consults a physician, much of the treatment depends on the patient's efforts. If he doesn't stay in bed, as ordered, or doesn't do the prescribed exercises, then nothing a doctor can do truly helps.

Any health consumer should be able to find information about the back and back care programs.

Of course, self-help must be approached intelligently. A person should guard against determining too much for himself if a serious problem is suspected. For instance, the wrong kinds of self-prescribed exercises can make a disk problem worse.

Perhaps self-help is best applied in learning basic posture and body mechanics to maintain back health.

YMCA EXERCISE PROGRAM

More than 200,000 people have enrolled in the classes of "The Y's Way to a Healthy Back" given at 2000 YMCAs located across the United States. The national program has been in operation since 1976 and still attracts full classes of students eager to alleviate their back problems.

The course offers six weeks of classes, meeting twice weekly. Participants, limited to 15, are taught a program of 18 exercises, including relaxation and limbering routines. Students also are expected to do exercises at home.

The classes also are offered to employee groups at industrial plants and at police and fire stations.

A survey of participants reveals 65 percent experienced good to excellent results.

Class fees for the course are moderate.

YOGA

Hatha yoga, the kind of yoga that would most benefit a back patient, calls for using your body to explore where you tighten up in daily routines. The purpose is to get away

Yoga to relax

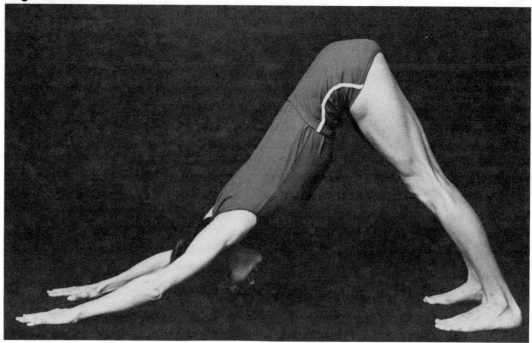

Yoga teaches a balance in the body between strengthening and stretching.

from the inevitable contracting against life and to be free to choose when not to tighten up.

At the moment there's a renaissance in hatha yoga because of the teachings of an Indian instructor, B.K.S. Iyengar, who has written a book entitled, "Light on Yoga."

His method calls for anatomically correct movements based on spinal alignment. His philosophy also has been followed by other yoga teachers.

All the poses are designed so the spine is always elongated. A key point is the belief that people don't know how to place their pelvis, considered important because the position of the pelvis affects what's going on with the spine.

Hatha yoga also teaches a balance in the body between strengthening and stretching.

One of the greatest gifts of yoga to some back sufferers is that it teaches relaxation. Many back patients have tense, Type-A personalities, so this is an important aid in helping them overcome back problems.

NINE:

TROUBLESHOOTING: SYMPTOMS OF BACK INJURY

Even physicians, with all their expertise, often are hard-pressed to diagnose a back problem accurately. The layman who wants to make a self-diagnosis is even more at a disadvantage.

However, the following list of symptoms will give you some clues as to your problem. As a general rule, the closer the pain is to the center of the back, the less severe the problem. Be concerned, though, if pain radiates from your back down the leg or if there's numbness or tingling in either the feet or the hands. These are signals of nerve impairment.

IF YOU FEEL:	IT MIGHT BE:
pain in your neck and numbness and tingling in your hands	cervical spondylosis
pain when bending backward	a facet joint problem
pain when bending forward	a disk problem
pain in the back, radiating down the sciatic nerve in the leg	a herniated disk
back pain at night that goes away after light exercises	ankylosing spondylitis
a sharp pain in one place in your spine, and you are 60 or more	osteoporosis
a backache and have a temperature of 100° or above	influenza or a kidney infection
pain in your back, as well as in other joints	osteoarthritis
pain in your back and inflamed eyes	ankylosing spondylitis
painful and stiff neck after receiving a severe jolt in the past day or so	whiplash injury
a severe pain in your neck and shooting pains in your shoulders or arms when you move your head	a herniated disk in your neck
difficulty in controlling your arm or leg muscles following an injury	spinal cord injury
a stiff neck when you awaken, although it was fine when you went to bed	acute torticollis
pain in the back between the ribs and hips, possibly accompanied by abdominal tenderness	a kidney problem

IF YOU FEEL:	IT MIGHT BE:
pain in the back above the lumbar region that can often be relieved by taking antacids	peptic ulcer
pain in the back, relieved by leaning forward, accompanied by gastric symptoms	problems with your pancreas
lower abdominal or sacral discomfort, accompanied by a vaginal discharge or by a relationship to menstruation	a gynecological disease
severe pain in the back following an accident or fall onto the buttocks	spinal fracture
severe progressive pain in the back in older patient; if you're older and have a history of malignancy, pain accompanied by spinal tenderness	cancerous tumor on the spine
lower-back pain after heavy lifting or unusually heavy labor	muscle strain
back pain intensified by coughing or sneezing	spinal stenosis

TEN:

BASIC BACK CARE FOR EVERYBODY

A person who has a painful back quickly develops the kind of posture that would be the envy of physical therapists everywhere. He sits up straight; he won't lean over a sink to brush his teeth because the back hurts so badly. In other words, he makes all the postural moves he should have made before he got hurt. The right posture might have prevented him from having a back problem.

There are basic rules everyone should follow for back health. They are recommended for both the person with a healthy back and the veteran back patient who wishes to avoid a recurrence of pain.

The exercises are simple and can be easily integrated into your life. Indeed, they should be practiced until they become automatic.

POSTURE

Of basic importance to back health is good posture, which sets the foundation for other movements. Often people stand with either a too-straight spine or an excessive swayback, particularly if pot bellies pull their stomachs down.

In a correct standing posture, the center of gravity should fall through the ear, the tip of the shoulder, the middle of the hip, behind the knee and through the ankle.

This position does not create a military, ramrod-straight posture but a relaxed, natural stance, with an acceptable amount of curve in the lower back.

Correct standing posture

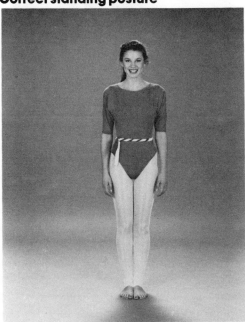

The center of gravity when standing correctly falls through the ear, the tip of the shoulder, the middle of the hip, behind the knee and through the ankle.

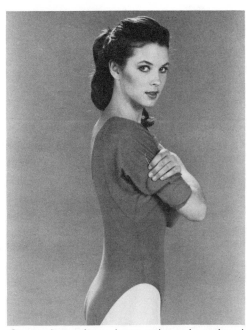

Correct posture is a relaxed, natural stance, with an acceptable amount of curve in the lower back.

73

The position of the head is equally important. Too often, people let their heads hang forward and down, compressing the spine. You should hold your head upright and the chin tucked back, flattening the curve of the neck. You want a curve in the lumbar spine but not in the cervical region.

SITTING

Sitting may be even more important in back health than good posture in standing. Many back problems stem from incorrect sitting and, in a nation where sitting is a way of life, from prolonged sitting.

The followers of the Robin McKenzie philosophy believe that the lumbar curve should be maintained while sitting. They advise putting a lumbar cushion or a rolled-up towel on the chair's back to aid in maintaining the lower-back curve. Otherwise, they

Correct sitting posture

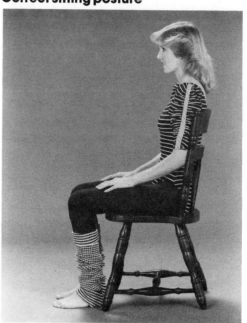

Robin McKenzie believes you must learn how to make a curve in the lower back while sitting and maintain that curve.

contend, the person will slouch into a rounded-back position, which is not good for the back. The supportive roll towel should be about three to four inches in diameter and may be partly filled with foam rubber.

In order to learn how to sit properly, McKenzie has said people must learn how to make a curve (lordosis) in the lower back while sitting, and to keep that curve while sitting for long periods.

Here is a suggested exercise: sit on a stool or bench, and alternately move your back from a slouch to an accentuated arch — stomach protruding, shoulders back. The movement takes you from the worst to the best sitting position. Once aware of the difference, you may then master sitting in a relaxed, good posture with a lower-back curve just short of the extreme.

Not everyone believes the use of a lumbar roll is necessary for good sitting posture. Some physicians advocate sitting in a firm chair with buttocks and back resting against the back of the chair.

Ideally, the back of the chair should be at about a 120 degree angle from the seat. Most rocking chairs are ideal for maintaining a correct posture because they allow for this angle in the back.

Although a firm cushion may not be needed to support the curve in the lower back, soft cushions are not advised. They allow your back to become rounded which should be avoided.

Here is the proper way to get out of a chair: Tighten your abdominal muscles and buttocks as you rise and use your arms and legs so that back motion isn't necessary. Avoid sitting with the legs extended in front of you. Sit with your shoulders straight and your head held high.

Sitting in a good position isn't enough to avoid back problems. Remember, sitting increases pressure on the spine, even under the best conditions. Always interrupt sitting for a few moments every hour; take a break and walk around. You'll give your back a brief rest. It's also a good idea to do a backward bend from the waist, with your hands placed at the small of your back. This stretch helps realign your spine after sitting. Taking a break from sitting is especially important while driving, because most automobile seats are bad for your back.

SLEEPING

When you're asleep, you don't know what position you're in. But you can at least put the odds in your favor by going to sleep in a position that's good for your back.

You should be sleeping in a bed with a firm mattress. However, the mattress shouldn't be so hard it's uncomfortable. For a firmer mattress, it often helps to slip a bed board, usually a rectangle of sturdy plywood, between the mattress and bed springs.

The two preferred sleeping positions are:

— Sleeping flat on your back with a small roll under the curve of the lower back to maintain the lordosis.

— Sleeping on your side with the top leg bent at the knee and the bottom leg straight. If desired, you can place a pillow under your chest to support your body.

Correct sleeping #2

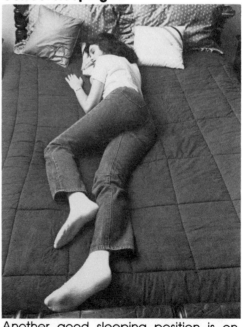

Correct sleeping #1

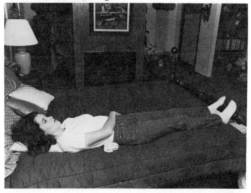

Sleeping flat on your back with a small roll under the curve of the lower back is recommended.

Another good sleeping position is on your side with the top leg bent at the knee and the bottom leg straight.

As with sitting, it's important to get in and out of bed properly. Don't just sit up from a lying position. Instead, roll onto your side to the edge of the bed, tighten your abdomen and push up — using your arms — to a sitting position as you slip your legs over the edge of the bed.

Getting out of bed

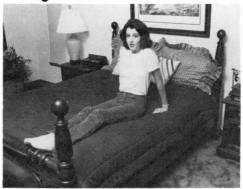

It's important to get out of bed properly–supporting your back. First, tighten your abdomen and push up–using your arms–to a sitting position.

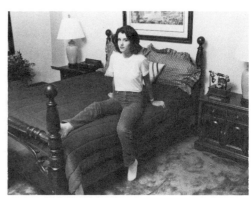

Then slip one leg at a time over the edge of the bed to the floor.

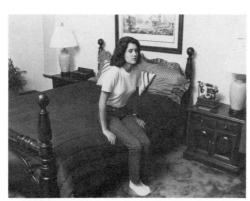

When both feet are together on the floor and you are sitting on the edge of the bed, push up with your arms.

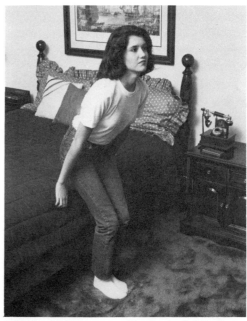

Be sure to keep your back straight when standing up.

LIFTING

We all lift or carry objects day in and day out. Improper lifting can either set off pain in your lower back immediately or over a longer period can cause severe chronic back trouble.

A basic principle in correct lifting is to have the object you want to lift close to your center of gravity. With the object close to you there's less danger of a back injury.

Here's how it's done. Stand directly over the object to be lifted; keeping your back straight, squat down in front of the object. Now lift, using the strength of the muscles in your legs and groin rather than your back.

Kinetic lifting

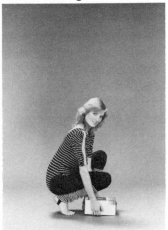 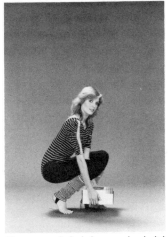 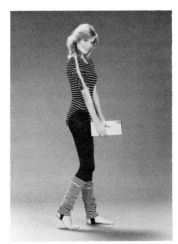

The kinetic technique: feet about 20 inches apart, one foot behind object, the other foot beside object pointing in direction of move.

Then, maintaining a straight back, start lifting.

Your back should be straight when the object is under control.

If you want to lift with one hand an object such as a pail or a suitcase, bend down so one knee is on the ground and the other bent in front of your body for balance. Keep the load near your body and don't bend your back as you use your leg muscles to rise and lift the object.

If you're carrying two suitcases or packages, the weight should be balanced so that your body is not pulled sideways, which increases lateral pressure on the back.

Another way to lift is called the kinetic technique. Thought by some to be the best way of lifting, it is taught to employees in many industries. If follows almost the same pattern as the straight-back lift with the object close to the body, the back straight, the chin in, a good grip on the object and arms close to the body.

Where the kinetic technique differs is in the position of the feet. They should be about 20 inches apart with one foot behind the object and the other beside the object and pointing in the direction in which it is to be moved. This position gives a broader base for the lifting motion which helps in maintaining stability and balance. By pointing the foot in the direction of travel, it isn't necessary to twist the spine when the object is lifted; you merely move the rear foot.

Care should be taken in reaching for things on high shelves. It's much better for your back if you use a stool or stepladder, especially if the object you're lifting is heavy.

OVERWEIGHT

Lifting may cause or aggravate back problems by exerting pressure on the spine. But how about being overweight?

Those extra pounds are a heavy load on the spine even though they may be distributed evenly over the body, although they usually aren't. Think about the potbelly that hangs over the obese man's belt. The potbelly is equivalent to lead shot tied around his stomach. Even worse, the weight is positioned so that it pulls the spine into an excessive curve. Here's a bad combination of swayback and excess pressure. Neither is good for the back.

One physician has estimated that 10 pounds of extra weight on the abdomen converts to 100 pounds of weight putting pressure on disks in the back. As the belly pushes out, the buttocks push back to offset the excess weight in front, accentuating the normal curve.

Pregnant women experience the same problem as the man with the potbelly, and it becomes especially acute in the last months of pregnancy.

One of the best recommendations for the potbellied person with back pain is to lose some weight. And in general the abdominal muscles should be strengthened to help hold the spine and stomach properly.

CLOTHES

High-heeled shoes may be sexy-looking but they don't help your back. That's because high heels tilt the pelvis and force the spine out of alignment. On the other hand, shoes that put the heel lower than the ball of the foot aren't good either. They may distort the proper position of the body.

A low or medium heel is best, and it should be firm enough to give sufficient support. Otherwise, it's too easy to slide or trip and wrench your back.

Purses can cause problems too, particularly for the woman who carries a heavy shoulder bag. Constantly carrying a heavy bag over your shoulder causes a lateral pressure on the spine. It's better to lighten the load or divide it into two bags, perhaps a purse and a tote bag.

The ardent photographer who travels around the world with a heavy camera bag over his shoulder also should take note. He may get good photos but there's an increased risk for hurting his back. If it's not possible to divide the load, at least switch the bag from shoulder to shoulder occasionally.

Here's another style note: Stay away from the skin-tight jeans that have been popular recently. They act just like girdles by propping up abdominal muscles, but will weaken muscles in the long run.

ELEVEN:

YOUR BACK AND YOUR LIFE

AT WORK . . . IN THE PLANT

Sometimes your back is better off at work than at home. Many health-conscious companies are enrolling their employees in back schools or educating them through other programs in the proper way to use their backs. At the same time, companies are redesigning the work place to make it kinder to backs.

Industry's motivation may not be altruistic. Bad backs mean lost profits to industry. As much as $75 billion is lost annually in the United States because of sick time, workmen's compensation and disability payments.

The intelligent company realizes it is more economical to spend thousands of dollars for education than millions for providing medical care and disability support to an injured worker.

However, not all companies are that enlightened. Some don't realize basic measures such as teaching a warehouse worker to lift or changing the level of the workbench, may make a significant difference in the back health of their employees.

What's called "bench work" is often a problem area for bad backs. The problem arises when employees in a factory or assemblers in an electronics plant, for example, have to work standing at a bench or counter. If it's too low, the worker must bend over his work. Ideally, the counter should be high enough so the worker can stand upright with a straight back. It sometimes helps, too, if the worker places one foot on a low stool.

Lifting techniques were described in the previous chapter. Workers who must do heavy lifting daily should be especially careful about following proper lifting techniques. Sometimes it may help to wear a heavy gridle or corset to give added support to the stomach muscles. And strong leg and groin muscles are extremely important for those who lift heavy weights.

AT WORK . . . IN THE OFFICE

The white-collar worker has his problems too. The executive is just as prone to back problems as the secretary, perhaps more so. The secretary probably sits in a posture chair that places her in a reasonably good sitting position. The executive sinks into a soft, easy chair, his back immediately assuming a bad position. All office workers risk back problems because they sit so much. There's not much that can be done about the large amount of sitting, although it might be possible to stand while doing some tasks.

To avoid back problems, sit with a straight back. Don't cross your legs above the knee and don't sit with one leg bent and resting on the other knee. Neither position is good for your back. It's better to sit at your desk with feet flat on the floor, although crossing the ankles is also acceptable.

Don't let yourself slump into a poor position when using a word processor or video display terminal. You've probably seen the position — buttocks at the edge of the chair

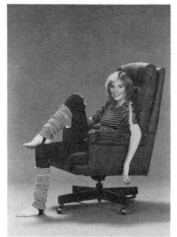

Many executives develop poor posture sitting in big, soft chairs.

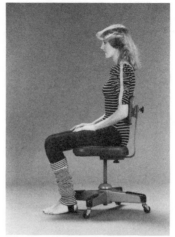

Chairs of many clerical workers encourage good sitting position.

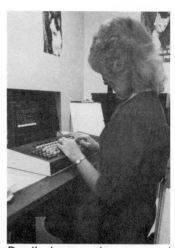

Don't slump using a word processor.

and the back in a slouch. Not only is this terrible posture for the lower back, but it strains the head and neck, too.

Another pointer for using a word processor: Place the material you're reading or copying so you needn't keep turning or lifting your head to see it.

If you wear bifocals, continually moving your head up and down to adjust your sight can cause strain, particularly if you have arthritis in your neck.

AT WORK . . . IN THE HOME

Any person who does a lot of housework will tell you that the work schedule is as full at home as it is for a factory worker. If you're working around the house, you have to follow the same rules of working and lifting as does the industrial worker.

For example, see that the counter where you work is at the correct height and stand before it using proper posture. Use correct lifting techniques. Check how you remove food from the oven. Most likely, you curve your back and bend over. Instead of doing this, do a version of a deep-knee bend to bring yourself level with the oven, remove the

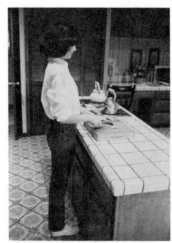

Make sure the kitchen counter is at a comfortable height for good posture while working.

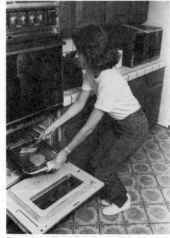

Do a modified deep-knee bend to bring yourself level with the oven when removing food.

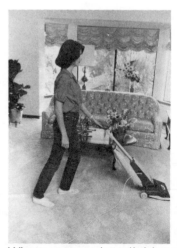

When vacuuming, tighten your abdominal muscles and keep your knees bent.

food, and then lift using your legs. To get something out of a lower cupboard, kneel on one leg with the other leg bent in front of you.

Vacuuming is a job that can strain even a strong back. Tighten your abdominal muscles while pushing the vacuum cleaner and keep your knees bent. Any bend should come from the hips and not from the spine.

Try to develop a rhythm of movement in whatever you're doing. If vacuuming or sweeping, push first with your right side, then with your left. The same principle applies to all repetitive movement, whether cleaning windows or scrubbing clothes.

Encourage children to pick up their toys and everyone to pick up their clothes so that you won't have to lift as often. When you do have to pick up something, remember to do it correctly by bending the knees, not the back.

Making a bed is bad for most people's backs, especially those who have a history of back problems. The bed is usually too low for their height so they have to bend over when making it.

One solution, highly recommended for people who have had many histories of back problems, is to kneel down beside the bed and make the bed from that position, even though it makes the job harder. If you're the average person with no serious back problems, standing and bending over to make the bed isn't going to ruin your back. Just remember to keep the back straight and to tighten your abdominal muscles. This reduces the stress on the back.

Stress should be kept to a minimum, and that means emotional as well as muscular stress. Don't overwork and get caught up in an "I've got to hurry and finish this job" feeling. Stay relaxed and take frequent short breaks. It's good for your morale and for your back.

IN PREGNANCY AND CHILD CARE

Pregnancy is a time when backaches may become more common, particularly in the last months when the abdomen is extended. The weight of the fetus pulls the spine into

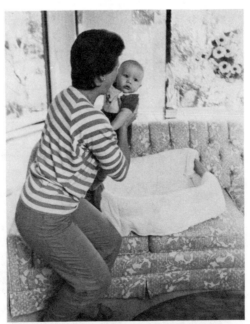

When lifting a baby, keep your back as straight as possible, tighten your abdominal muscles and tuck your buttocks.

an unnatural curve, putting pressure on the spinal column. A woman who starts out in pregnancy with strong stomach muscles will have fewer back problems. Every effort should be made to keep your posture as correct as possible to counteract the excessive swayback.

After the baby is born, more problems may arise. The stomach muscles are usually weak after the pregnancy, yet the new mother has the added chore of caring for a baby. This means a lot of lifting and bending, both conducive to poor back health.

Keep in mind the following: It helps to have the table where you change diapers and dress the baby at a height that allows you to stand with a straight back. When lifting the baby from the crib, remember the principles of correct lifting. Keep your back as straight as possible, tighten your abdominal muscles and tuck your buttocks. It's also a good idea to start an exercise routine to regain physical fitness as soon as possible.

IN THE CAR

If you're not at work or at home, chances are you're in your car. We live in a mobile society. A businessman drives to appointments and a housewife chauffeurs children to and from school and to recreational or entertainment activities. Then on Sundays the whole family often goes out for a leisurely drive.

All that sitting in a car seat wreaks havoc with the back. Just consider this scenario: At a meeting of fundraisers for charitable foundations, all of whom had recently spent a lot of time in their cars, the work at hand was forgotten as everyone began discussing his back problems and what he did to alleviate them. One fundraiser had even resorted to using her clipboard as a support for her back.

As you might imagine, truck drivers suffer back pains because of their long hours at the wheel. But they often have an advantage. An awareness of the importance of proper seats has developed in the trucking industry and the seats of a commercial truck are probably better designed than those of a luxury American car.

Luxury doesn't have any relationship to proper seating in an automobile. An expensive and elegant Italian sports car, the Lamborghini, was described in one rating of car seats as having "dreadful hammock-type seats."

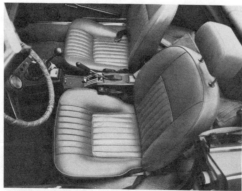

The ideal car seat for maintaining good back position is a firm seat with a downward tilt to the bottom section and a slight backward tilt to the seat back.

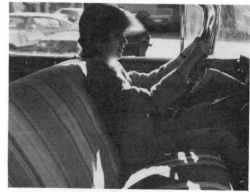

The back sinks into a curve on soft, "bench" car seats, putting stress on the disks.

Sports car seats like the Lamborghini's are totally unsuited for maintaining good back posture. If the car seat is too low, the driver's legs are held nearly straight, putting increased pressure on the back.

On soft, cushiony car seats, the back sinks into a C-chaped curve that causes stress on the disks. The ideal car seat is firm, with a downward inclination in the seat part that accommodates the buttocks and a slight backward tilt to the back of the seat to provide support for the upper back.

To get into the car with the least back strain, first put your buttocks on the seat, then swing your legs in.

Even with the best of seats — and few automobiles win prizes in that regard — you always should take frequent breaks on a long trip. Sitting for hours in a stressful position is hazardous to your back.

Getting in a car

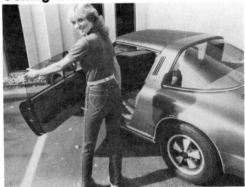

There is a proper way to get into any type of automobile.

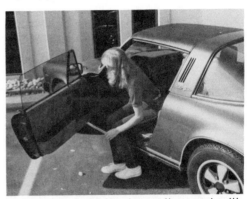

First, put your buttocks on the seat with your legs still outside the car on the ground.

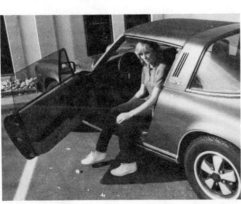

Once seated, swing your legs into the car and turn to rest against the back of the seat.

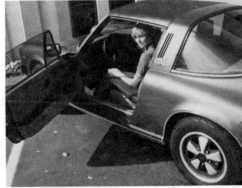

When you're completely inside the car, make sure the seat is adjusted correctly and move around a bit until you feel comfortable.

As a side note: If you're ever called upon to push a car, do it correctly. Instead of facing it and pushing with your arms, back up to it and push with your buttocks and the muscles of your legs.

IN AN AIRPLANE

Airplane seats are usually better designed than auto seats, so that's a help. Even then, long flights can be hard on a back. The best way to cope is to move about as frequently as possible. Walk up and down the aisles by going to the bathroom even if you don't have to. You might even try one of the backward bending movements recommended in Chapter 10, if you're not too self-conscious.

Once at your destination, you're often faced with sleeping on thick, lumpy pillows and a sagging, soft mattress or on your friend's narrow couch. It's a sleeping arrangement that's almost sure to start your day with a stiff neck and an aching back.

Some people with bad backs like to carry a small, flat pillow in their suitcases. It doesn't take much room and can make nights on the trip much more comfortable.

If your back is sensitive and you need a firm bed at a motel, ask the manager to supply a bed board. Even a second-class hotel in a small Italian town was able to provide me with one on request. It's also possible to carry a folding board along with you. If necessary, move the mattress to the floor and sleep there. It may be a little uncomfortable, but so is a back problem.

AT PLAY

If play for you means the singles bars and cocktail parties, have a fine time. Just be sure to stand in the correct posture, and walk around the room frequently.

Play also means going to watch recreational activities like football and baseball games. At these you usually sit uncomfortably on narrow bleachers for several hours. There's not much you can do about it, either. Just try to sit in a correct position, maintaining a curve in your lower back. At every break in the action, take a break yourself. Walk to the food concession stand. The movement will relax your back if nothing else.

Active sports, although they can be hazardous to your back because of injury, help build muscle strength, which is indirectly good for the back. But the advantage of health and fitness far outweighs the lesser chance of back injury from exercising.

Walking is the ideal exercise for back-problem sufferers. Often a physician, in addition to prescribing a set of corrective exercises, will suggest a short walk at lunch time or after work. And jogging and running should present no problems as long as they are done correctly. The correct running posture will vary from individual to individual, depending on the amount of normal lordosis or curvature of the lower back, the amount of changes in the spine from age and how the joints have adjusted in the lower back to the upright position. You shouldn't run with your chest sticking out in an exaggerated pose, nor with your trunk bent far forward, unless you're running up a steep grade. Both put undue stress on the spine.

Because of the popularity of jogging and running, Dr. Arthur H. White, director of the St. Mary's Spine Center and founder of the California Back School in San Francisco, made a thorough study of the subject. He says that any back patient who can walk fast can jog, but that the jogger should shorten his stride and bend his knees more as a way of producing less jarring.

In addition, the jogger should focus on holding a pelvic tilt and keeping his abdominal muscles tightened. At first this style might seem uncomfortable, but the jogger soon becomes accustomed to it. However, he should break into this posture gradually.

Running is more of a strain on the back because the stride is longer, the back curve is extended and the jarring greater, White found. The runner will have to test his limits to find out how much he can do without pain. There are many ways to reduce the jarring from running and jogging. Running on a soft surface like dirt or grass helps, as do good running shoes. Uneven ground and hilly terrain can cause more jarring.

White advises that the jogger learn to listen to the sound of his feet hitting the ground. With a fast walk or shuffle there's little or no sound, but as the jogger overstrides or becomes tired, the sound of his feet hitting the ground becomes louder and louder. That's a sign to alter his style of jogging or to stop.

Warm-up and stretching exercises are important with running and jogging, as with other sports.

Some sports cause very few back problems. Sports medicine physicians see few golfers in their practice. Golf doesn't cause problems unless there is an uncontrolled follow-through that may put pressure on a facet joint or disk. Some players find the bending and twisting is almost like a manipulation that's helpful to their backs.

Tennis is a satisfactory sport for players with a history of back problems as long as the game is not fiercely competitive. A high, hard serve may overextend your back. This risk can be avoided by lowering the point at which the ball contacts the racket.

Swimming is a good exercise for back patients because the buoyancy of the water takes pressure off the back. However, the back patient is cautioned against overdoing it, such as concentrating on the butterfly stroke or holding a paddle board in front of him and kicking his feet. Both of these activities may put too much pressure on the patients back.

Bicycling is an ideal sport for the person who has spinal stenosis, a narrowing of the vertebral canal. But don't ride hunched over. Adjust the handlebars so you are leaning forward with a straight back. Patients with spinal stenosis are often more comfortable in the upright position with a slight forward lean.

To sum up, a back patient can do an amazing number of sports activities as long as he isn't suffering an acute attack of pain and as long as he doesn't overdo it. The important point to remember in all sports is to keep your body in proper position — your back straight, abdominal muscles tight and your buttocks tucked.

AND SEX

There's no reason why back problems should interfere with a satisfying sex life except perhaps for the times when a patient is in real pain. Some people use a backache just as they do a headache, as an excuse for getting out of doing something they don't want to do. Wives or husbands, either consciously or subconsciously, latch onto a slipped disk problem as a plausible alibi for not being affectionate. Of course, interest in sex can vanish if the activity causes pain.

A safe way for a back patient to have sex is to be the passive partner, lying on the back in a pelvic tilt position, with the abdominal muscles tightened and the buttocks tucked. Lying on the side is another possibility.

Most minor disk and facet joint injuries heal sufficiently in a week or two to allow sexual activity. In more serious cases, you should check with your physician.

IS A WATER BED BEST?

Many times, once a person realizes he has a chronic back problem, the first thing he does is go out and buy a water bed. He's heard the rumors: A water bed is just what an aching back needs.

One doctor says that a water bed, as long as it's heated, has the potential for keeping the back warm, which might offer some advantage. Most doctors don't take a firm stand against water beds and usually give a patient a go-ahead to get one. But after the initial attachment, the patient's romance with his water bed usually ends. A water bed is hard to climb in and out of, so it puts added stress on the back. Water beds also are harder to make up than an ordinary bed.

A physical therapist agrees water beds are fine as long as they're firm. But they're better if only one person is sleeping in them.

The therapist has a water bed but is thinking of switching to a regular mattress. He weighs 195 pounds and his wife weighs 112 pounds. It makes for a very lopsided sleeping situation.

TWELVE:

THE BACK IN YOUTH AND AGE

Middle age is the time when back problems start showing up in earnest as chronic misuse and the years catch up with people. However, the young and the elderly have their own special problems.

THE YOUNG BACK

The young are mostly free of back problems except for those caused by congenital defects.

One childhood back problem is spina bifida, the condition in which the lower part of the spine that helps protect the spinal cord fails to develop properly. This may appear only as a small dimple in the back or it may be very severe, resulting in nerve damage that may mean the child will need special braces and crutches or a wheelchair to move around.

Another disorder, one that strikes most often at young girls, is scoliosis, a lateral curvature of the spine. The cause of the curvature may be due to a congenital abnormality of the spine, to paralysis or weakness of the back muscles or to an abnormal growth of the spine associated with dwarfism.

Most cases have no known cause, otherwise called idiopathic scoliosis. The severity can range from being so slight the curvature isn't noticed to being severe enough to cause recurrent chest infections and shortness of breath.

Many schools offer screening programs to test for scoliosis and it's important to diagnose the problem early because it may get worse. Corrective measures include doing exercises to strengthen the muscles or wearing a specially shaped corset until the defect is corrected.

Adolescents may suffer from Scheuermann's disease, sometimes called "adolescent round back." In this disorder, which is a common cause for backaches among teen-agers, unexplained growth changes in the thoracic vertebrae give them a wedge-shaped form. This increases the normal curvature in the upper back. During the active stage of the disorder, which can last from two to five years, there may be some pain. The problem is self-limiting, and is not considered serious although it possibly could cause an unattractive deformity.

Restriction of activity and back muscle exercises are normally the only treatment required. In more severe cases, the teen-ager may need bed rest and a spinal brace. In some cases, a spinal fusion may be necessary.

Another back disorder of the young is spondylolisthesis. The ailment involves the forward displacement of a vertebra in the lower back caused by a bony defect between the vertebra and the arch that encloses the spinal canal. It may be a congenital condition or may have developed early in life. The slippage is caused by degeneration of a disk next to the vertebra.

The disorder can exist without showing any symptoms and may be discovered accidentally during a routine physical checkup. Symptoms, if they occur, are lower-back pain and pain in the leg.

The treatment is the same as for disk degeneration. If there are no symptoms, nothing need be done and the young person can lead a normal life.

The British back expert, James Cyriax, believes spondylolisthesis is caused by repeated strains on the lowest two lumbar vertebrae when the infant is about a year old.

Stress fractures occur between the two halves of the vertebral arch but cause no problem until some time during adolescence when, after years of tension, the defect enlarges. The vertebra becomes longer and eventually projects in front of the one below it. An unstable joint forms between these two vertebrae and a disk lesion results.

Cyriax notes that not all people with spondylolisthesis have symptoms and, if they do, the symptoms are not always caused by disk lesions. However, he says symptoms are usually present.

Stress fractures that set off spondylolisthesis are blamed by Cyriax on the repeated bumps an infant takes in the first year of life. The baby, too young to walk, moves about while seated, with each shove bouncing his buttocks along the floor. When a baby first learns to walk, his legs give way and he repeatedly falls on his seat. These repeated stresses are considered the main cause in a condition that is present in about 4 percent of all patients with backache.

Cyriax advises discouraging babies from pushing themselves along while seated, and to see that they crawl untilthey learn to walk. They also should wear padded diapers to cushion their falls. The doctor approves of the various "walkers" that enable a baby to stay upright and push himself along on rollers.

Back problems may appear in a youngster because one leg is shorter than the other. This condition throws the spine out of balance and can cause back pain. The treatment calls for inserting a corrective lift to be worn at all times in the shoe of the shorter leg.

The only truly reliable way to measure leg length discrepancy is to take an X-ray of the pelvis and both legs of the patient while he is standing.

A wise and caring parent will try to protect his child against future back problems by teaching him some of the same basic body posture mechanics that are used by adults. Be conscious of your child's posture and try to encourage proper standing and sitting habits. Even if a child wants to flop down on the couch to watch television, his back position can be improved by tucking a cushion behind his back to maintain the lower-back curve.

Teach your child how to lift objects. He may pick up the technique unconsciously from watching you do it. If not, give him a lesson in lifting. It's certainly as important to his future health as the regular physical exams and dental checkups.

THE OLD BACK

Visualize the pristine new back of the young — the vertebrae all shiny and strong and the disks full and cushiony. Then visualize the backbone of an old person. Degenerative changes have overtaken the vertebrae. They are knobby and may have bony growths.

The disks have lost much of their bounce. The jellylike center is drying out and there may be cracks or tears through the outer walls of the disks. This disk shrinkage may cause a noticeable loss in height.

No wonder the old have back problems. Their spines were designed for a briefer life span. Longevity has outstripped evolution.

Despite the aging process many old people don't have problems. X-rays may show a lot of wear and tear but either they have used their bodies well or have maintained fitness. They don't suffer the back pain that plagues some of their younger friends.

One disorder that causes back problems for older people is spinal stenosis; bony growths on the spine, combined with the shrinking disks, cause pressure on nerve roots and consequently back pain. Some doctors believe the condition is present to some degree in everyone older than 70, although it is a condition that was rarely recognized five years ago. Although the nerves are affected, there usually is no sensory or motor loss in the legs. However, there may be severe pain in the buttocks and thighs.

An estimated 80 percent of the patients with this condition recover well if they cooperate in losing weight, exercising and correcting their posture to reduce excessive swayback.

Another common problem in the elderly back is osteoporosis, or thinning of the bone. In this condition, the bones lose mass and become thin and brittle, susceptible to tiny stress fractures. The condition may show up with symptoms of band-line pain going around the upper body, because of pinched nerves. More common back pain symptoms also may be present.

Osteoporosis can cause the "hunchback" of old age, because of a partial collapse of the vertebrae. The disintegration is more apparent in the front than the rear of the vertebrae, creating a wedge-shape.

Presently, most physicians believe osteoporosis, which is most common in postmenopausal women, can be prevented by taking estrogen hormones for the first eight years after menopause.

Good exercise habits and proper nutrition are important in keeping the bones strong.

Arthritic changes can affect the elderly person's back. The arthritis may affect the facet joints at the sides of the vertebrae, making the back stiff and painful. Dr. Walter M. Bortz, a specialist in geriatrics at the Palo Alto Medical Foundation, sees old people with backaches daily in his practice.

"Almost all the time they are due to poor muscle tone, degenerative arthritis and poor posture," he says. "Lots of old folks get the stoops because they generally don't pay attention to keeping their spines in correct alignment."

He finds that the older patients will describe pain in functional terms — they have trouble getting out of a chair or out of a bathtub — instead of complaining about the pain itself.

Rather than attempting a complicated diagnostic workup for these common complaints, Bortz tries a triad of treatment, prescribing heat, rest and something for pain.

"Pain begets spasm which begets pain," Bortz says.

A heating pad or a hot bath helps to relieve the spasm and undo the pain cycle. Often, Bortz says, older people get into bad posture habits to escape pain. He will start them on aspirin or Tylenol, then move on to non-steroid anti-inflammatory drugs if they appear in order.

Another reason that causes patients to come in is upper-back problems. Commonly, the patient will complain about poor circulation in his hands, or muscle spasms in the neck. The same general principles of rest, heat and pain relief apply here. Bortz may also prescribe gentle stretching exercises and sometimes a soft neck collar to take pressure off the neck.

THIRTEEN:

MENTAL ASPECTS OF BACK PAIN

A major hindrance in diagnosing back pain is pinning down an exact description of a patient's pain. One doctor explains, "It's difficult to ascertain where the pain is located and it's difficult to interpret what it means. Equally difficult is the problem of deciding what is the significance of the pain to the patient.

"I'm sure all doctors see patients with the same injury or illness and some of them slough it off and may not even come to the doctor," he continues. "Others are in agony from presumably the same degree of pain. The back is a good example of the extremes of pain sensation. I don't know whether it's the personality of the patient or whether there's something about backs in our society that fill people with dread, despite the fact it's a common problem . . . or maybe because it's a common problem."

Whatever the reason, a patient's back pain often has a strong psychological element. Perhaps it's because of the feeling of vulnerability a back problem can engender. You're going along normally and then a minor action — reaching for something in the car or picking up a piece of paper — suddenly leaves you bent over with an agonizingly painful locked back. If that happens once, you reason it can happen again. From then on you feel like you're walking a tight wire and any twinge of pain may be magnified.

On the negative side, a dull backache that lasts for a long time can begin to dominate your life. You're always uncomfortable, always conscious that you're hurting; you begin to restrict your movements. No wonder depression can take over and pain become a way of life.

To make matters worse, back pain often strikes during the difficult years when you realize age is creeping up on you. The younger people at work are beginning to make you feel superfluous, and you feel stymied in your job. This is the age when the children have left home, which can make a mother feel useless and unwanted.

It's painful to reconcile yourself to growing old. You may feel the same inside, but a sudden glance at the mirror and you catch a glimpse of the gray hair and wrinkles. When back problems enter the picture, it's another affirmation that you are, indeed, falling apart. The feeling is intensified because you're not likely to get any assurance from your doctor that your problem is a clear-cut one, easily treated. Instead, you may get vague explanations like "I think it may be a disk that's slipped out of place . . . we'll try bed rest for a while." There you are in bed with nothing to occupy your mind except the pain in your back and the fear that you'll end up being incapacitated for life.

The emotional aspects of back problems may explain why in many cases of back pain nothing seems to help. A laminectomy performed to correct a disk problem might not relieve the pain, even though the surgery itself was a success.

Doctors have reasoned for a long time that a major portion of lower-back pain is linked to the patient's mind rather than to organic problems of the spine. Back specialists estimate that in 80 percent of the back cases where there does not appear to be a definite cause for the problem, pain takes the form of stress, worry and other emotional states.

Some patients even seem to have a subconscious need to hang on to their back pains. They may use the pain as an excuse to drop out of life or as a way to get attention or affection. Doctors are becoming more aware of this use of pain to get sympathy. In cases where doctors feel it is a problem, they will counsel the family to avoid sympathizing too much with the individual's complaints. Instead, they suggest giving the patient more support and attention when he acts in more positive ways toward overcoming back pain.

Boredom and depression are emotions that may be turned into lower-back pain. The woman home alone all day with no children to keep her busy may fill her day — and night — by creating, subconsciously of course, a good case of back pain. Then she can become occupied with going to the doctor and can use it to get attention from her family.

Depression can accompany back pain. It's a classic "Which came first, the chicken or the egg?" situation. Did the depression start after the person developed a back problem that restricted his activity or did he start out by being depressed and is using the back pain as an overt expression of that depression?

Many people won't outrightly admit, "I'm depressed," but it's easy for them to say, "My back hurts."

Many people use the same strategy, but they choose a different ailment to express it, such as a headache or stomach pains. One description given of this emotionally based back pain is that "it's just a tension headache that has slipped down the back."

Doctors are beginning to think there is a typical back pain personality. They describe people in this category as hard-driving but lacking in self-confidence. They are likely to repress anger and to avoid conflicts.

Whatever the underlying factors, physicians realize they must view the patient with the knowledge that the back and the mind are intertwined. It's not enough to just treat the back; the doctor also must be aware of what's going on in the patient's mind.

Of course, not all patients have such definite psychological dimensions to their back problems. As with other medical problems, a back patient can view his problem as merely a physical illness, receive treatment and be cured. Even though the back problem may recur, he is objective enough about his illness to associate the new pain with a physical cause. He will resume exercises or become more careful about watching his body mechanics.

But there's a hard core of chronic back patients whose pain seemingly cannot be resolved by the traditional treatments. Psychological factors may be accountable. The patient may be unconsciously magnifying the pain or aggravating his condition. He may need a psychologist as much or more than he needs an orthopedic surgeon.

Studying Chronic Pain

In reaction to an awareness of this need, the medical community has put a new focus on understanding chronic pain and searching for ways to alleviate it. As yet, there isn't a complete understanding of how pain is transmitted. Recently a nerve pathway was discovered that leads from the brain stem to the spinal cord. It apparently acts to control pain transmission and seems to be activated by a variety of things, including psychological factors and drugs.

Another area of research has focused on endorphin and enkephalin polypeptides, which bind to opiate receptors in the brain and raise the pain threshold. It's still unclear how this occurs, but it has significant promise in developing clues to ways to control pain. The polypeptides are morphinelike substances that are formed naturally within the brain and control the normal experience of pain.

Until the recent breakthrough in research, it was thought that a pain stimulus, such as a burn or cut, would stimulate special receptors in the skin that would convey a message along the nerves right up to the brain, producing the sensation of pain.

This was a partial explanation of how pain was transmitted, but there were unanswered questions. Why did some people have a greater sensitivity to pain than others? Why would the same individual sometimes be able to brush away pain when at other times the same degree of pain would be felt much more severely? For example, soldiers in a battle or a boxer in a fight might receive severe injuries but not be aware of the pain at the moment.

The simple pathway theory of pain transmission couldn't explain these incongruities. There seemed to be some other action within the brain that influenced the experience of pain. The discovery of the endorphins and enkephalins filled in some of those gaps. It was discovered that these brain substances served in the same manner as morphine to block pain. Evidently, the transmission of pain involves not only the nerve pathways but the brain itself; which has a mechanism for releasing polypeptides that will affect how the pain is perceived. All the answers aren't in yet, by any means, but the knowledge is expanding rapidly.

Researchers now know there are fibers in the spinal cord that will stimulate preferentially the brain's pain-controlling center and prevent the sensation of pain. There also are fibers that descend from the pain-suppression center of the brain down the spinal cord that control the transmission of impulses between the nerves and the spinal cord itself. There are receptors in the spinal cord that respond to endorphins of the same sort as in the brain.

The new knowledge also explains why a placebo is often effective in relieving pain, sometimes as effective as an accepted medication. A placebo is a preparation containing no medicine that is given for its psychological effect. Of course, the patient is not told that it is a placebo.

Just because a person responds to a placebo doesn't mean he faked the pain. Research at the University of California in San Francisco has shown that about one-third of the pain patients who respond to a placebo show an increase in the level of endorphin released by their brains.

Physicians who are aware of this knowledge may try to integrate the idea into their treatment of back patients. They may not go as far as prescribing placebos, but they will make a greater effort to communicate a positive attitude to the patient. Giving the patient hope and an expectation that treatment will cure the pain may influence the cure.

Research is underway now exploring whether endorphins can be given by mouth and whether they might be useful in alleviating chronic back pain. Trials have been made with synthetic endorphins and they have been demonstrated to be capable of producing relief of pain when injected around the spinal cord.

Until that research is completed, physicians are using other techniques in their efforts to help the back patient whose pain appears to some degree to be the result of a psychological factor.

Chronic pain clinics. These clinics have quickly expanded around the nation, devoted not only to the back patient but to any patient who has a history of chronic pain that can't be attributed to organic causes.

In some instances, the standbys of bed rest, exercise and medication are used to help control the pain. But these are being prescribed from a more knowledgeable position. Before, a physician might prescribe a medication that tended to suppress endorphins and promote depression. Now there is a broader selection of medications and a better understanding of what they can accomplish.

However, physicians are increasingly cautious about the overuse of drugs, particularly in cases of chronic pain. A study at the Mayo Clinic in Minnesota revealed that 65 percent of 144 chronic pain patients had some type of drug dependency problem.

Physicians have learned that when people take narcotics for a prolonged period they often confuse their drug dependency with their pain. When the narcotic wears off, they feel a need for more of the drug. The tendency is to label that feeling as pain, rather than as the drug dependency it really is.

Drugs. Among the new medications used are a wide range of non-steroidal anti-inflammatory drugs that reduce inflammation in a manner similar to that of corticosteroids but without their side effects. The new medications of this type can be taken less frequently than aspirin and cause fewer gastrointestinal problems. For reasons that are unclear, one form of these drugs may relieve a patient's pain where another one won't. Doctors switch around until they find the most effective one for that particular patient.

However, some side effects are recorded with a few of these medications, including the risk of bone-marrow toxicity, which may limit their long-term use.

Other Treatments. Physicians and pain clinics also are using mechanical means to reduce pain. One technique is biofeedback, a form of behavior therapy in which the person can learn to control his responses. Acupuncture, a treatment from the Far East, holds promise as a way to relieve pain that has a psychological component. Some practitioners think acupuncture also stimulates release of endorphins and enkephalins.

Another technique that may be used to relieve chronic back pain is called transcutaneous electrical nerve stimulation (TENS). This has gained popularity in the past 10 years. The technique is based on a principle that dates back to the third century when gout pain was treated by putting patients in water to be stung by electric rays or torpedo fish.

In TENS, as it's used today, electrodes are taped to the skin of the lower back, adjacent to the painful zone or over a nearby sensory nerve. The electrodes are connected to a small portable generating unit. The patient can generate mild electrical impulses when he wishes and can vary the intensity of the impulses and the time of the stimulation. TENS has been used to treat a variety of chronic pain, including lower-back pain. In chronic cases, it appears to be successful 40 percent of the time, about half the rate of success for the technique in acute-pain problems.

The pulses are felt as pricking sensations and the controls can be adjusted to provide the most comfortable level. The stimulator is worn on a belt or carried in a pocket and the patient can go about his normal activities, switching on the apparatus when the need arises. The unit produces minute amounts of electric current, so there is no danger of any burns.

Some patients get remarkable relief from pain using the TENS technique, with the relief lasting as long as several days. A false stimulator, like a placebo, has given the same good results in some situations. TENS is favored because it is a non-invasive technique that has little potential for harming the patient.

Other techniques for dealing with the most severe cases of chronic back pain can be more drastic. Previously, doctors whose back patients suffered from chronic pain were more willing to perform surgery, but this has changed with the realization often the surgery doesn't stop the pain.

Unsuccessful surgeries of that type created a category of back patient called the ''lower-back cripple,'' someone who had two or more laminectomies to correct disk problems but who was still suffering pain. Estimates are that surgeons now operate on only about five percent of the lower-back pain patients who would have been considered good surgery candidates in the past.

This change is seen as a reaction to the experience in past years of successful surgery correcting the disk problem but failing to relieve chronic pain. As a consequence, today surgery is predicated on stricter criteria and with a sensitivity to whether the pain is caused by psychological factors.

However, a surgical procedure designed to relieve chronic pain has been used with some success. It is called "cingulotomy," a psychosurgical procedure. Some physicians have reported using cingulotomy successfully to relieve chronic lower-back pain but other physicians question the value of the procedure; they argue that a long term follow-up demonstrates the pain often recurs.

ON-THE-JOB INJURIES

A type of back patient not mentioned before is the person injured on the job or in an accident who stands to gain financially from his back pain, whether through workmen's compensation, social security or insurance disability payments.

Are the claims valid or not? Again, it's hard to be certain, given the vague nature of back problems.

One trick doctors can use to trip up malingerers is to test them this way: The patient is asked to kneel on a stool, lean over and try to touch the floor. This is something even

The "bend-over test"

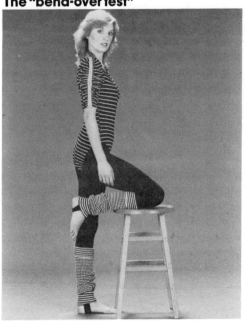

One test many doctors use to make sure a patient really has a physical back problem is kneeling with one leg on a stool.

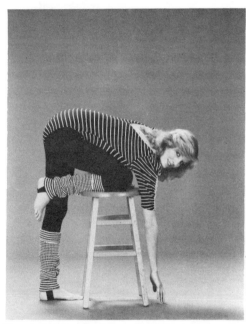

Then the patient is asked to lean over and try to touch the floor. Ironically, even back sufferers can usually do it.

someone with a severe disk problem can do but the malingerer more often than not refuses to try on grounds the pain would be too great.

The idea of people faking back problems to win financial gain is so common there's a term used to describe it — "compensation neurosis." The term is applied when doctors and lawyers claim the patient won't get better until he has received his compensation. Then the symptoms will disappear without treatment. The truth of this argument hasn't been proved. A study of patients with persistent headaches in a similar situation failed to find any effect of compensation on the outcome of headache pain.

The persistent pain following a back injury may be because of the actual damage or psychological factors, but it's an oversimplification to say the patient is just after money. The person may be seeking compensation, not in dollars, but in sympathy and concern from his family and friends. There's more than one kind of payoff for having back pain.

FOURTEEN:

PREVENTING BACK PAIN

Being able to cure back problems once they develop would be wonderful, but it would be even better to not suffer the back problem in the first place.

That's not as farfetched as it sounds. Prevention of at least most of the common backaches that plague people is possible by following simple rules.

For years, no one thought much about proper care of the back. People waited until they were faced with pain, went to the doctor and then tried, with more or less diligence, to keep the pain from recurring. They often failed. In recent years, however, much new knowledge about the back has developed. There's better understanding of how the spine works, of the effects of stress and emotional attitudes and the importance of body mechanics. More importantly, there's a recognition that following the rules of back care can prevent many back problems from developing.

Preventing recurrence of back problems is essential, too. Many people may not even be aware of their backs until they've had one episode of pain. Then they want to learn how to avoid a repeat episode.

By its nature, lower-back pain is self-limiting. Statistics have shown that 44 percent of patients with lower-back pain are better in one week, 86 percent within one month, and 92 percent within two months.

If a person had just one episode of back pain that got better by itself, back problems wouldn't be the burden they are.

Although each episode may be self-limiting, the pain recurs and the recurrences tend to become more severe with each successive attack. A patient who learns techniques to relieve the first episode of back pain has learned not only how to stop pain, but how to prevent a recurrence.

Rules to Prevent Problems

The basic rules for prevention of back problems are as follows.

1) Maintain proper posture. Stand tall and straight with a normal lower-back curve and with your body in balance.

2) Avoid prolonged sitting. Move about frequently. During breaks, realign your spine by placing your hands at the small of your back and bend backward.

3) Be careful about lifting. Keep the object to be lifted close to you, bend your knees and lower yourself to pick it up, rather than stooping over with your legs straight. It's a simple maneuver. Wouldn't any person choose to do that instead of risking back pain, sessions of bed rest and perhaps even surgery?

4) Teach prevention to the children. Pediatricians say preventing health problems in children is one of their most important roles. As with adults, prevention of back problems in children is easy.

Just see that your child sits, stands and lifts correctly. Even better, do these things correctly yourself. Your child will imitate your moves.

5) Develop good exercise habits. Back health is helped by strong abdominal and leg muscles and by flexible quadriceps and Achilles tendons.

Public Interest

Evidence of public interest in preventing back problems is quite strong. Stores specializing in chairs and other posture aids that promote back health are popular. Even drug stores are advertising posture cushions. The trend is a healthy one. The more public attention focused on back health, the more incentive there is for people to follow good habits.

Exercising and Relaxing

The YMCA, which has helped thousands through its national "The Y's Way to a Healthy Back" program, recognizes the need for preventive medicine. A pilot program has been developed by the YMCA in Palo Alto, Calif., focusing on the prevention of back problems. It is designed for those people who haven't experienced problems yet but who are interested in learning more about their backs. Classes are held on location at businesses and industries.

The program includes three sessions, each lasting an hour or an hour and a half. The first session concentrates on the anatomy of the spine and mechanics of injury. The instructor says that people will follow the rules of back health more diligently if they understand the reasons behind them.

The second session touches on the person's way of life and the workplace, back exercises and treatment options in the event of an injury.

The final session focuses on the middle and upper back and neck, which are more prone to problems caused by stress.

The program integrates many of the newer ideas that have been advanced in back care by such men as Robin McKenzie, the New Zealand physiotherapist who has had a dramatic impact on the back community.

Participants in the YMCA course are encouraged to follow a routine consisting of five exercises. They are:

1. Lie flat on your back with your hands down at your side and with knees bent, feet flat on the floor. Bring your knees up to your chest, hold for 15 seconds, and return to starting position.

2. Lie on your back on the floor with both legs bent, heels on the floor. Using your hands, bring one leg up to your chest, return to starting position and then bring other leg up. Do not hold the knee to chest position but just touch chest and then return to starting position.

3. Lie on your back, hands crossed over your chest and heels on the floor. Take a deep breath, and curl your chin to your chest as you begin to exhale. Lift your shoulders and upper back off the floor, and hold momentarily. When you run out of breath, inhale, then uncurl and return to starting position. The exercise should be done very slowly.

4. Lie on your stomach with your hands clasped behind your back. Lift your head so you're looking straight ahead. Then at the same time, lift your head and shoulders and your feet off the floor. Hold that position for five to 15 seconds, then return to the starting position.

5. Lie on your stomach with your hands at chest level, palms on the floor. Then press up, extending your elbows and curving your back. Hold for five to 15 seconds, before returning to starting position.

Doing these exercises will take only a few minutes a day. The routine is kept simple so that it will be easier for people to fit it into their busy routines.

Much harder than doing exercises is finding the self-discipline to avoid stress and to relax to avoid triggering back pain. The Alexander Technique is one popular modern day relaxation method. The Alexander Technique, which embodies principles on the proper use of the body, was developed by Australian Matthias Alexander. He calls for a relaxed, serene approach to life.

Edward Avak of Menlo Park, Calif., director of one of the three approved schools in the Alexander Technique in the United States, lives by that philosophy. However, he says he realizes it is not an easy accomplishment.

"I would say to a person, 'Cultivate an ability not to rush,' " he urges. "I think rushing probably takes one of the heaviest tolls in terms of misuse of the back, physically as well as mentally."

He adds, "You just can't say to someone who's stressed and hurried, 'Slow down.' You not only have to convey to him the importance of slowing down but also the idea that slowing down is not something he can just turn on or off.

"It has to be an ongoing struggle he can work through to make a fundamental change in his life."

Avak also advises people to pay attention to what they are doing at the moment, rather than thinking of what they are going to be doing over the next 20 hours. He says he thinks people are more liable to hurt themselves and injure their backs if their minds are not on what they're doing.

"If you treat slowing down and good back care as simple, trivial things, people often try a bit and then give up," he says. "They think it should be easy to do and are discouraged on finding it isn't."

The same reaction applies to adopting the simple rules of back health outlined here. You'll probably read these words of advice and, for a day or two, conscientiously watch how you stand. You may do the exercises a few times. But unless you make a real commitment, you probably won't be very faithful about following the rules of prevention.

You may get off easy and be one of the lucky ones who goes through life without a back problem. Then again, you may twist around to pick up something and, "Wham!" there goes your back. As you bend over, agonized with pain, you'll undoubtedly think, "I should have done my exercises."

Remember, it's never too late to start. The same rules that help to prevent back problems can help avoid a recurrence of the problem.

FIFTEEN:

QUESTIONS AND ANSWERS

I'm expecting a baby in five months and realize that my big, heavy stomach will throw my back out of position. It's uncomfortable enough just being pregnant; I don't want a backache too. Is there anything I can do?

Back pain is common in pregnancy because the weight of the uterus stretches the muscles of the abdominal walls and pulls the spine, creating an exaggerated lordosis or swayback in the lower back. One way to reduce the problem is to watch your weight. Don't add too many excess pounds beyond what's needed to produce a healthy infant. A support girdle may help relieve the strain and low-heeled shoes are recommended.

If my back starts hurting, how can I judge whether it's serious and if I should rush immediately to the doctor?

A rule of thumb is that the nearer the pain is to the center of the back, the less serious it is. Be concerned if the pain radiates down your leg, especially if there is numbness or tingling in the toes. That indicates pressure on your sciatic nerve, possibly because of a ruptured disk.

I'm a pharmaceutical salesman and have to carry around a heavy bag of samples and literature as I visit physicians' offices. I realize this load isn't good for my back but what do I do about it?

If possible, try to divide the weight equally into two packages for carrying. You might put the samples in one case and the literature in another. Or you might change the side you carry your case on frequently, and take rest stops to give your back a chance to recuperate.

I hear about all the workers who fake back problems so they can collect workmen's compensation. Isn't there any way to expose them?

Some doctors subject suspected malingerers to this test: They ask them to kneel on a stool and lean over and try to touch the floor. Usually even someone with a severe disk problem can do that, but the faker may refuse to try, complaining it would hurt too much.

Although there aren't any conclusive figures, there aren't as many back-pain fakers as people think. There may not be any apparent organic reason for the pain, but because of psychological factors, the pain is real to them.

My garden is the joy of my life, but since I've developed back problems it's a torment to try to do gardening. Is there any way I can protect my back and yet enjoy my hobby?

The best way to do weeding is on your hands and knees, maintaining a straight back as you work. This gets tiring, so some gardeners like to rest their chests on a low stool covered with a cushion. It may look ridiculous but it helps.

For raking or hoeing, move the tool handle with the arms and keep your body upright. Push a wheelbarrow or lawn mower with the handles held behind the thighs so that the arms are held slightly backward, arching the back.

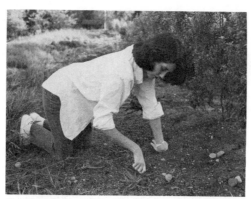

The best way to weed a garden for your back's sake is on your hands and knees, maintaining a straight back as you work.

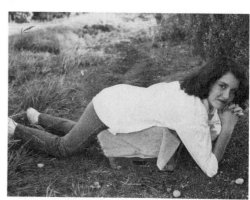

The best way to rest while weeding is to rest your chest on some sort of low stool or box covered with a cushion or towel.

And remember the cardinal rule. Take frequent breaks to realign your back by doing exercises.

I'd like to guard the health of my back but my life is crowded and harried enough as it is. I don't have time for exercises. Is there anything I can do that will not be so time-consuming?

Yes. Just be conscious of your posture, both standing and sitting. Good posture, and that means standing straight but with a natural curve in the lower back, is one of the keys to preventing back trouble.

I've had recurring problems with back pain and am worried that may mean I'll have to give up my favorite sport, tennis. My back bothers me after a game. Should I stop playing?

You shouldn't have to give up tennis if you pay careful attention to how you play. By using correct body mechanics, even back patients can participate in most sports.

Slow your game and play doubles instead of singles. Watch your posture and don't try to go after the low, difficult shots even if it means losing a point.

You may have to change your serve, too. Don't reach as high to hit the ball and don't hit it as hard. It may not be the same game you used to play but you can still enjoy tennis.

My elderly mother is depressed because her back is bothering her and she feels her life is being limited. Is there anything I can do?

See that she makes an appointment with a physician who is interested in back problems and aware of the special problems of old age. There's no reason for your mother to suffer from back pain. There are treatments, such as medication and heat, that can help. It might be useful, too, for your mother to take antidepressant medicine to break her out of the pain/depression cycle.

After all I've read about the dangers of estrogen hormones, I've now heard that estrogens may help prevent osteoporosis or thinning of the bones. I certainly want to avoid this disease but I'm afraid of taking hormones after all the warnings they might cause cancer. What should I do?

This is a subject you should discuss with your doctor. He can advise you individually on the safety of taking estrogen hormones; presently, the estrogen therapy appears to be making a comeback. Perhaps he can measure your bone mass and tell if you have reason for concern about osteoporosis. Perhaps exercise and good nutrition will be enough to protect you.

Everyone says you should do sit-ups to strengthen your abdominal muscles but I've heard some ways of doing them are wrong. What's the correct way?

Exercise experts now realize the old-fashioned way of doing sit-ups — sitting up and touching your toes — may create problems in your back. The sit-up favored now is this isometric version: Lie on your back with knees bent and feet on the floor. Arms can be folded over your chest. Lift your head and trunk just until your shoulders are clear of the floor. Hold that position for a bit, then relax.

It seems like everybody is either weightlifting or working out on the Nautilus machines. Are they safe for my back?

Most of the Nautilus machines are designed with a slanted backrest, which gives them good support for your spine. The seats have straps to hold the back and pelvis in a safe position.

Lifting free weights shouldn't present a problem either, as long as you have firm support for your back. As with the Nautilus machines, while lifting weights, tighten the abdominal muscles and tuck your buttocks. As always, remember not to overdo. Build your strength gradually.

I spend a lot of time on the phone each day, and my posture isn't the best then. What suggestions do you have?

The tendency, if you're sitting with a phone to your ear, is to slouch in your chair and to hold your neck at an angle. Neither is very conducive to back health.

Use good posture while phoning just as when doing anything else. Hold your head upright with the chin tucked in and keep your back straight except for the normal lower-back curve. Sometimes you may be able to relax and phone at the same time by standing and leaning your back against the wall. Bend your knees, with your feet away from the wall and your back flat against the wall.

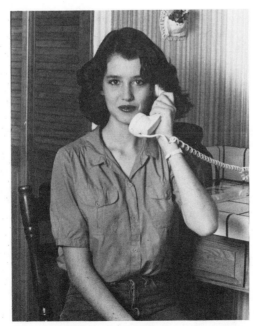

Good posture for talking on the telephone is to hold your head upright with chin tucked in and your back straight except for the normal lower-back curve.

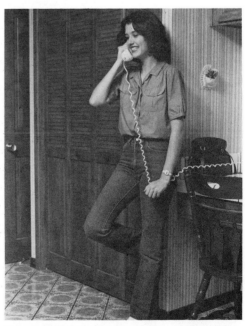

If you want to relax while on the telephone, try standing and leaning your back against a wall.

What's the best way to be sure my child grows up with a healthy back?

Encourage your child to sit, stand and lift properly but, most importantly, do all these things yourself. As with any other learning experience, it's not very convincing if your attitude is: Do what I say, not what I do. Children learn best by imitation.

The podiatrist fitted me with orthotics because I was having a problem with my feet. But as soon as I started using the orthotics, my back began hurting. Why?

Your back hurt because the orthotics changed the position of your body and you began using your back muscles in a different way, even using different muscles. Break into wearing orthotics gradually so your muscles have a chance to adapt.

I feel that I've developed a dependency on drugs because of the pain I've endured with my back. Does this happen often?

Drug dependency is definitely a problem, particularly when back pain becomes chronic. Once a chemical dependency is established, the patient may confuse the need for another ''fix'' with pain.

Use medication sparingly, only during acute attacks of pain and search for ways to avoid the recurrence of back problems.

SIXTEEN:

TOMORROW'S REMEDIES AND TREATMENTS

America's commercial side *is* paying increasing attention to the back. For example, chair manufacturers are making products with improved back support. Back support pillows are also a popular item. It would be even better, of course, if all furniture was designed with back health in mind. That is something we have to look forward to. More and more people are becoming aware of the ubiquity of back problems and there's a widening realization that back problems aren't inevitable.

Back problems, as we've learned, can be prevented by proper posture and movements. The slogan, "Once a back patient, always a back patient," no longer rings true. Recurrence of back pain can be prevented if the patient follows the rules of back health.

Much more is known now about how the spine functions and why and how the vertebrae, the disks and facet joints can cause problems. There's also a greater understanding of the roles of muscles, not just in the back but in the legs and thighs and stomach.

Technological developments in medicine have contributed to this knowledge. The CAT scan, by making it possible to get an X-ray of the soft tissues of the back, has done much to help physicians understand what goes wrong with a disk. A new form of treatment called chemonucleolysis, using an enzyme from the papaya called chymopapain, makes it possible for the patient with a herniated disk to avoid surgery.

Despite the explosion of knowledge, medical experts don't think we're in the Golden Age of back care yet. There is still controversy about the most effective kinds of treatment for back problems. The arguments will continue until there is more exact knowledge about why a treatment works and on which patient it should be used. Research and clinical trials are needed to test the different therapies, to show how they work and the most efficient ways to apply them.

A clearer understanding of what causes back pain is needed. Although there's more comprehension now of back problems than ever before, there is still a large category of complaints in which there's no apparent organic reason why the patient feels pain. More research is needed to gain knowledge about the role of endorphins and enkephalins in controlling chronic pain, along with a better understanding of how pain is transmitted.

The psychological aspects of back problems need to be explored. How much pain is tied in to emotional factors and how can a patient's psychological health be improved?

Another dream of doctors is to find a substance that could be injected into intervertebral disks that would restore them to their full, cushiony health. Attempts have been made along this line, using silicone and other substances, but as yet nothing has worked.

More work needs to be done in the area of prevention, too. Industry and business are becoming aware of the problems and are developing health-education programs for their employees. More needs to be done along these lines.

The programs must be expanded to include office and assembly line workers. After all, they suffer from back problems as much as the factory worker.

Back education programs should be included in schools as a part of the child's basic education. Even a kindergarten child can learn the proper way to lift, thus establishing a good habit early in life. Teen-agers learning to drive an automobile should be taught the proper way to sit in a car seat, and the need to avoid prolonged sitting without taking a break.

All these objectives can be accomplished, and will be when there is enough public demand for them. With all that needs to be done, the picture is bright for back patients. There have been great advances in the medical community's ability to help people with back problems. Coupled with that are the advances in understanding how an individual can help himself to improved back health.

Even if your back is hurting as you read this, take heart. There's help out there and more on the way.

BIBLIOGRAPHY

The American Medical Association, *Family Medical Guide*. New York: Random House, 1982.

Associated Press, ''Half-Dozen Studies Explore Osteoporosis.'' August, 1983.

Barlow, Wilfred. *The Alexander Technique*. New York: Warner Books, 1973.

Better Homes and Gardens Books, *New Family Medical Guide*. Des Moines, Iowa: Meredith Corp., 1982.

Cornfeld, Joe. ''Getting Aggressive About Conservative Therapy for Back Pain.'' *Medical World News*. July 5, 1982.

Cyriax, James. *The Slipped Disc*. Epping, Essex, England: Gower Press, second edition, 1975.

Deyo, M.D. MPH, Richard A. ''Conservative Therapy for Low Back Pain.'' *Journal of the American Medical Association*. Aug. 26, 1983.

Ehni, Dr. George. ''Seeking the Hidden Flaw.'' *Spine*. Vol. 6, No. 4, 1981.

Friedmann, Dr. Lawrence W. and Lawrence Galton. *Freedom From Backaches*. New York: Pocket Books, 1976.

Gray, Henry. *Gray's Anatomy*. Philadelphia: W.B. Saunders, 36th edition, 1980.

Gunby, Phil. ''Chymopapain: Tropical Tree to Surgical Suite'' and ''What is Intradiscal Therapy, Anyway?'' *Journal of the American Medical Association*. March 4, 1983.

Hogan, Brian J. ''Seating Design can Cause Lower Back Problems.'' *Design News*. Sept. 13, 1982.

Jayson, Malcolm I.V. *Back Pain — The Facts*. New York: Oxford University Press: 1981.

Kraus, Dr. Hans. *Backache, Stress and Tension: Cause, Prevention and Treatment*. New York: Simon and Schuster, 1965.

Kraus, Dr. Hans, Alexander Melleby and Dr. Sawnie R. Gaston. Back Pain Correction and Prevention.'' *New York State Journal of Medicine*. July, 1977.

Livingston, Dr. Michael M. *Back Aid — Your Guide to Care of the Back*. Philadelphia: George F. Stickley Co.

Medical World News, ''CT Scanning Hailed as Guide to Dramatically Better Back Surgery.'' July 19, 1982.

Medical World News, ''Postmenopausal Estrogen Therapy Appears to be Making a Comeback.'' July 27, 1983.

McKenzie, Robin A. *The Lumbar Spine, Mechanical Diagnosis and Diagnosis and Therapy*. Waikanae, New Zealand: Spinal Publications, 1981.

McKenzie, Robin A. *Treat Your Own Back*. Waikanae, New Zealand: Spinal Publications, 1980.

BIBLIOGRAPHY

Prudden, Bonnie. *Pain Erasure the Bonnie Prudden Way.* New York: M. Evans and Co., Inc., 1980.

Time Magazine, "That Aching Back!" July 14, 1980.

Trubo, Richard and Charles D. Bankhead. "Pain, Assembling the Pieces of a Complex Puzzle." *Medical World News.* Aug. 8, 1983.

Webb, Penny, M.S. "Back to Self Care?" *Physiotherapy.* Sept. 1982.

White, Dr. Arthur H. *Back School and Other Conservative Approaches to Low Back Pain.* St. Louis: The C.V. Mosby Co., 1983.

White, Dr. Augustus A. III and Stephen L. Gordon, Ph.D. "Synopsis: Workshop on Idiopathic Low-Back Pain." *Spine.* Vol. 7, No. 2., 1982.

INDEX

ABOUT THE AUTHOR

Mary T. Fortney, a staff writer for the *"Peninsula Times Tribune,"* Palo Alto, Calif., first became interested in medicine when working part-time for a San Francisco physician while attending the University of California in Berkeley.

Her job was to do the billing, but after the financial book work was completed, she'd delve into the doctor's library of medical books.

Medical writing, however, didn't come until later. After graduation from the University of Oregon, she worked in San Francisco as managing editor of the *"Daily Commercial News,"* a business daily; managing editor of the *"Pacific Shipper,"* a maritime weekly, and as a financial writer with the *"San Francisco Examiner."*

She left San Francisco to join the *"Peninsula Times Tribune,"* then the *"Palo Alto Times."* Seeing the need for coverage of all the medical stories generated by a lively medical community that included the Palo Alto Medical Foundation and Stanford University Medical Center, she volunteered for the assignment. She currently covers both medical and general news assignments.

A series of articles on medical treatment of children born with congenital heart defects won her a first-place newspaper writing prize from the American Academy of Pediatrics.

The Palo Alto Medical Foundation for Health Care, Research and Education was established in 1981 as a non-profit, charitable institution integrating the highest caliber of medical care, basic scientific research and health and medical education.

The Foundation's three divisions, their goals and purposes are:

• The *Health Care Division* is staffed by the 145 physicians of the Palo Alto Clinic, a physician partnership, and nearly 600 nurses, medical receptionists and support staff. This division strives to provide complete, high-quality medical care at the lowest possible cost.

• The *Research Institute* is built upon more than 30 years of internationally acclaimed achievement by the Palo Alto Medical Research Foundation.

Now the Institute, as the research division of the Medical Foundation, works on basic scientific questions of worldwide importance, in areas such as immunology and infectious diseases, bio-engineering, physiology, microbiology, genetics and medical economics.

• The *Education Division* plays an increasingly important role in both health education for the public and medical education for physicians, nurses, medical receptionists and others in the medical field.

With the spiraling costs of medical care, it becomes even more important for each person to take a more active role in maintaining good health. Effective education and health promotion is the key to giving people the information and skills they need to assure their well-being.

The Foundation is located in Palo Alto, Calif., approximately 30 miles south of San Francisco.